Healing Together

30 Stories of Personal Transformation Through Holistic Healing Modalities

Compiled By:
The Community for Holistic
Integration

PAVE PRESS 81-2447736,
408 W. Maple St., Dallastown, PA 17313
pavepress1@gmail.com

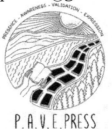

P. A. V. E. PRESS
ISBN 978-1-7334590-3-7
Library of Congress Control Number: 2020904752
April, 2020
Cover Art Jimmy Purkey
Printed in United States of America

*This book is not intended as a substitute for the advice of a medical professional. The reader is advised to regularly consult with a physician in matters relating his/her physical or mental health and particularly with respect to any symptoms that may require medical attention.

CHI does not specifically represent or endorse any products, brands, or spiritual viewpoints mentioned nor guarantee any one holistic modality over another. Methods, tools, and spiritual views are shared solely at the discretion of individual authors. Please research all available options before choosing a course. A directory of CHI Practitioners of various modalities can be explored at www.chiweavers.com

Table of Contents

FOREWARD 1
CHI President Stacey Duckworth

A Letter from Our CHI Board Secretary 5
Erin Shrader CHI Board Secretary

About CHI 7
www.chiweavers.com

My Journey Back to Me 9
Judy Forder 18

Painting for My Life 20
Jimmy Purkey 23

A Journey of Transformation 25
Peg Zimmerman 33

Making Sense of the Remnants 35
Worksheet: Pieces of Me 43
Kimber Bowers 44

Coming Back to Life 46
Erin Shrader 60

What Makes Your Heart Sing? 62
Linda Felch 66

A Fresh Approach to Personal Change 67
Pattie Craumer 73

Therapeutic Art 75
Louise Kemper 79

Select Poems 81
    Strong Women.. 82
    Healing... 83
    Reflections.. 85
    Quotes... 86
  ...Laile Wilson 86

My Four Truths of Reflexology 88
    Leslie Punt... 92

The Mirror: From Ashamed to Powerful 94
    Kerri Hample 98

For the Love of Reiki 100
    Katye Anna 104

Poems of Transition 106
    Flores Para Los Muertos.................................... 107
    Some Thing.. 110
    Hope 111
    A.N.I.. 113
    TransitionS for Every Body................................ 114

My Transition... 114
    Annabell Bonilla 119

The Key to Transformation 120
    John Stewart 124

My Journey from Health Helper to Holistic Health
Coach 126
    Rebecca Johnston.. 134

Gratitude Page 136
    Eleanor Justice

The Profound Healing Magic of a Feather and a
Flower.. 137
    Brandy Yavicoli 142

Second Chance Collar 144
    Clinton R. Chronister....................................... 151

How I Fully Recovered from
Complex PTSD 152
    Clinical EFT Basic Recipe..152
    Mindful Meditation..153
    9 Gamut Tapping...154
    Mary Kalbach 164

Gut Feeling 166
    Kerri Hample 172

Following The Stars..173
    Angie Whitsel...181

A Simple Shift 182
    Meditation for Acceptance....................................168
    Kimber Bowers 188

Resilience.. 189
    Denise VanBriggle 193

The Lotus Eater 195
    Communing With Ancestors Meditation....................185
    Michele Lefler 209

Collective Communication Empowers................. 211
    Erec Smith, Ph.D.. 219

Politics Lost: My Campaign for Office 220
    Stacey Duckworth 224

Prince Was Right 225
    Yoga Routine for Strength & Stamina.....................213
    Nicole Montanarelli...................................... 232

What Might Your Pets Have to Say?..................... 234
    Leslie Dull-Runkle.. 237

Mustard Stains and Crooked Tiaras.......................239
   Phyl Campbell...243

Trusting The Path 245
   Rachel Rosado- 254

Journal Prompts
To Help You Get The Most Out of This Book..........256

27 Things To Remember
On Your Healing Journey 263

Acknowledgements 266

Index i

FOREWARD
CHI President Stacey Duckworth

We should approach life doing what we know we can – not what we think we should.

Once upon a time, we had a really great idea — something so perfect it filled us with excitement and wonder. We couldn't wait to share our idea with someone else. Until we did. Unfortunately, as soon as the words left our mouths, we received negative reactions.

We heard, "Why would you want to do that?" We heard, "You'll never be able to do that." We saw head shakes of disappointment, felt and heard the laughter of derision. Our exciting, perfect, absolutely brilliant idea soured, becoming "stupid" or "a silly pipe dream" in an instant. Our happy world shattered. Sometimes we stopped ourselves even before we even shared the dream —deciding that miserable lives in society's acceptable boxes were easier to live with than rejection.

Most of us experience these feelings. Fear of failure makes us overthink the risks of asking for a raise or promotion, going back to school — and forget about leaving the working world we know for self-employment or creating something new. More often than not, we are told what we cannot and should not do, rather than being encouraged to nurture or explore what could be. The practicalities of life restrict us. Our responsibilities — our bills, our chores, our families, and our children — come first. They should take precedence — shouldn't they? Responsibilities require acknowledgement, attention, compassion, and care.

We love our families — especially our children. They didn't ask us to bring them into this world. They are not a burden to us, or they shouldn't be.

But what about those great ideas of ours? Those sparks that sneak up every once in a while, reminding us of more, nudging us in the direction of the what ifs? Don't those sparks deserve the same kindness and attention as our responsibilities do? Our children may grow up, but our responsibilities never go away. Why shouldn't we allow ourselves to dream bigger? To see the spark and follow through? If no one tried anything new, we wouldn't have washing machines (for clean wet clothes to mildew in when we forget about them).

What if — let's just say — as an experiment, we break the chains of normalcy? What if we explore the woulda - coulda – shouldas that lie just past our unending responsibilities? What if we actually approach life doing what we know we can rather than what we think we should? What if we allow the flame to flourish and give it a chance to speak?

Some of us spend years resigned to living lives that fit into the proverbial box. We present ourselves to society the way we are "supposed to be." We go through the motions that seem to fulfill all the roles and appease nearly everyone. Everyone but us. Until we reached our breaking point. Then maybe we shout, "enough is enough!" into the proverbial atmosphere. We tear out of the box that suffocates us and follow the sparks that ignite and inspire us.

As many CHI collaborators discuss in our meetings, CHI itself would not exist if the practitioners involved waited for the people around us to "get it." Outside our meetings and practices, there are still plenty of people who don't get us, don't trust us, feel threatened by us, or actively discourage us. However, because we move in spite of our fear, because we listen to our inner voices and follow our excited sparks, because we seek each other out and form a larger community of support, we are able to find what we've needed to become better versions of ourselves.

In this book, we find many stories of people just like us, people who have decided to live their lives exploring the what ifs. People who have found personal betterment and fulfillment along the way. As CHI collaborators, we will share our journeys and how braving daring moments exploring what could be changed our lives. Some may resonate more than others. But it is our hope that all will inspire us to rekindle flames within so we can live lives that excite us and bring us joy.

Stacey Duckworth

CHI President

A Letter from Our CHI Board Secretary
The Rebel Herbalist Erin Shrader

Dearest Reader,

Like a river in wintertime whose surface is frozen over but the deep waters continue to run onward toward the sea, our outer persona is often the hardened mask of who we should or ought to be while deep within there is a movement and a flow that carries us ever onward toward our truest self. If you have opened this book, then you certainly have also felt this flow within your own life. If we trust this current and pull up our oars (and our anchors!) we can be carried onward to what we cannot imagine.

My hope for this book is to act as a companion on this journey with you. I hope you will reflect on the joys and the pains of opening a life to depth, purpose and intimacy. When feeling the first flutters of this opening in our lives we can often feel alone, overwhelmed and even betrayed by the life we are living and the people we love and who love us. I hope you will find comfort in knowing that these feelings are shared by many. This is a time of great stirring and shifting for human beings on Earth. This time has been called "the Great Turning," "the Shift," "the Great Work," and many other names. We are waking up to our place in a story that is much bigger and grander than we have been led to believe.

I have spent my life trying to figure out what has happened to us, and to find ways to restore our hearts to their wholeness, and to remind people of their magnificence. I have been writing love letters for years, to all sorts of people. This book is our love letter to you.

I am honored to be on this journey with you. As Ram Dass reminds us, we are all just walking each other home.

In love,
Erin
Dover, PA
January 19, 2020

About CHI

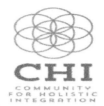

The Community for Holistic Integration is a grass roots movement to bring holistic wellness to our community through connection, education and integration.

Our mission is to connect holistic practitioners and practices located in Central PA, so that we may unify our causes to benefit one another in serving the most underserved and most needed areas of our community.

To educate the public on various holistic practices and modalities so that they may accept and appreciate incorporating holistic-minded practices into their lives without trepidation or hesitation due to unfamiliarity or misconception.

To integrate holistic practices into our society to benefit all community members so that they may experience the benefits associated with living holistically and respecting, recognizing and healing the mind, body and heart of each individual.

To uphold the values of integrity, kindness, personal freedoms, and respect while working towards unification of our community

The authors in this publication, all esteemed members of the CHI community, can be found in our directory along with other Central PA Holistic Practitioners at www.chiweavers.com

Together, we are bringing our community back to life!

"Don't ask what the world needs. Ask what makes you come alive and go do it. Because what the world needs is people who have come alive." ~Howard Thurman

My Journey Back to Me
Judy Forder

In order to share my healing journey through Reiki and other holistic modalities, I feel it is important to provide you with a little background and general understanding of how I accumulated the various masks that I have worked years to remove in an effort to show up as my true authentic self in every aspect of my life. Having done the inner work, I now understand that each mask was created out of a need for survival to cover/block an emotion and I honor each and every one. Don't worry, I'm not going to share about **all** of them, only the heaviest ones. Let's start at the beginning...

My name is Judy Forder. Born on December 10, 1969 to Richard L. Forder, Sr. and Doris Diane Forder. I've been told that my brother was disappointed I wasn't a boy but loved me anyway and my sister would never have her own room again but somehow managed to love me as well. I was the baby of the family for about four years, then came my little sister. Finally, I got to be a big sister and I loved it!!

Looking back, we were the average middle-class family and life was good.

My first day of kindergarten my mother took me to school in a pretty dress, tights and patent leather shoes. At the end of the day, my dress was filthy and my shoes were scuffed. Day two my mother tried again, and again I came home a mess. You see, recess was my absolute favorite thing about school. By my third day, Mom decided to let me be me and I wore shorts, shirt and sneakers to school. Perfect attire for recess, don't you think? As a result of my chosen sense of style and the fact that I played with the boys much more than the girls, I found myself labeled a ***"Tomboy."*** This label I wore proudly because I could beat most of the boys in my class at any athletic challenge as well as hold my own in a scuffle, if need be. Growing up one of four kids with multiple cousins, I had to learn to handle myself especially when fighting for that last fresh bagel that Grandma and Pop-pop brought from the deli on their way to the house. Life was good.

I was in third grade when life changed for me. I overheard my doctor tell my mother I was fat and should be put on a diet. In that moment I knew I was different and not in a good way. There was something wrong with me that needed to be fixed so that I would be "normal" and of "average weight." Let me introduce you to my mask of **Shame**. I looked at my body in the mirror with disgust and dreamed of being thin. As I mentioned, I was a very active kid, loving recess, riding my bike, climbing trees, playing football and whiffle ball with the other kids in my neighborhood. I ate what my mother gave me, but nothing seemed to change. Life was good... on the outside.

By the time I was in fifth grade I was learning that if I made jokes about my weight before other kids could, I would be seen as the funny fat kid and they would like me instead of tease me. If I said the terrible things first, in a joking way, then it wouldn't hurt as much, right? Introducing my mask of **Self-Deprecating Humor**. It didn't take long for me to learn that you could diffuse almost any situation with humor, and I became a master at it. Life was funny... on the outside.

Then came middle school. I went from a small elementary school where I had established myself as the funny fat, yet athletic, tomboy to a much larger school. A couple of months into the school year I gained the attention of a girl named Tammy. Tammy was not very nice to me, but I would do my best to joke my way out of every interaction. Then one day she approached me in the cafeteria and started picking on me. I finally reached my limit of her bullying. I stood up in front of what felt like 400 kids and challenged her to hit me. The next thing I know, my friend Michelle, was standing next to me. She told

Tammy, "You don't want to mess with Forder because she will kick your ass right here in front of everyone."

Michelle was hilarious in her own right and was able to diffuse the situation by cracking some joke and Tammy never bothered me again. In that moment, my reputation was cemented. As a result of her saying what she did, kids like Tammy left me alone, and if I was friends with someone, the bullies left them alone, too. Around this same time in my life, I overheard my brother telling my parents they didn't have to worry about me because I could take care of myself and everyone else for that matter. Welcome **The Protector**. Life was interesting...

The persona I had created carried me through high school pretty well. High school friends may have described me as outgoing, funny, confident, friends with almost everyone, and the life of the party. Life of the party because I had started drinking when I was around fifteen years old. I was hanging out with older kids and wanted to fit in, so not only did I drink but I worked very hard to drink the guys under the table. I am very grateful that it never became an issue and once I was serious about sports I no longer drank when I was in season. It was great training for college though!

It was in college when I discovered I was gay. Going to school to be a physical education teacher could have tipped me off, but we all learn at our own pace, right? This was in the early 90's and things were definitely not as open and accepting for the LGBTQ community as they are now. Hell, I didn't even know there was a community! Things finally made sense to me about how I had been feeling about relationships and what was expected of me. Fear had made me hide my new discovery from nearly everyone. I had a boyfriend and was just going to figure out how to make it work. Apply the mask of **Deception** and another layer of **Shame**. Life was even more interesting...

My mother was diagnosed with Lupus in the early 90s as well. Nearly nothing was known about Lupus then, so they treated her with massive amounts of steroids, which destroyed her body. In July of 1996, I lost my mom. My rock, the person who could always calm my storms was suddenly gone. I was lost, sad and angry. My parents were always very affectionate and the love they had for one another was obvious to everyone they met. My Dad had watched my mother suffer for years and that wore heavy on his heart. After losing her, he made the decision to take his life in a different direction. This caused a lot of hurt feelings and I felt fatherless as well as motherless. Apply the **Orphan**. Life sucked...

For the next six years I spent my weekends drinking, commiserating with my siblings and focusing on my anger toward my father and his new wife. To honor my mother and bring my siblings together, I attempted to duplicate a few of mom's signature recipes then have them and their families over for dinner. Our family was blessed to have my niece and eventually nephew provide us joy, love and laughter every time we were together. Their young innocent energy brought light to my otherwise very dark heart. I was a physical education teacher and coach at this time. Working with kids also brought my heart joy but gradually, the more closed off and numb I could make my heart, the easier it was to get through my day. I think I should mention that not long after my mother died, I came out to my family. They all knew already and were very loving and accepting, but the words were spoken, and it was made clear that my "roommate" was not just a roommate. I carried a tremendous amount of guilt because I'd never had a conversation with my mother about the "real" me. I came to learn she had spoken with my siblings about the possibility of me being gay and they said her only concern was my safety and it made her sad because she always thought I would be a great mom. Let's add **Guilt, Anger** and **Disappointment** to my collection of masks. Life was numb.

In the early 2000s, my girlfriend (who eventually became my wife) and I began talking about possibly having a baby together. We had been together for nine years and we both wanted to be mothers. A few out celebrities had started families and we thought we could too. In 2002, we decided to move forward and began the process. On

December 15, 2004 we were blessed with a beautiful, healthy baby girl. Just like many other first-time moms, my heart had no concept of unconditional love until that little life was placed in my arms. I was determined to be not only the perfect mom but the perfect lesbian mom. Apply the illusion of **Control**. Life was busy but good.

Eight years later, on December 5, 2012, I went for my first Reiki session thinking I would check it out to see if it would help my little sister who was suffering from chronic illness and pain. When I left the treatment room that day, I had no idea what happened, but I knew I needed more. I went home and within two hours contacted the Reiki practitioner and scheduled weekly appointments from now until whenever. I felt lighter. I felt hopeful. I realized that whenever anyone would ask me how I was doing I would respond with "Just working to get through the day!" And I meant it. I had a beautiful, smart funny little girl, a family who loved me, a partner who loved me and a job I enjoyed (for the most part). I found myself asking why my heart wasn't happy. Why couldn't I feel and accept all the love I had in my life? Life was confusing.

After each weekly session, my life got lighter and lighter. I was accessing all the emotions I had not allowed myself to express or work through, the heaviest being grief. I had never allowed myself to grieve the loss of my mother, or my grandparents, for that matter. Opening that door lead to anger, which required forgiveness. Forgiveness for all the people who had hurt me and caused me pain or made me feel less than, unworthy, ugly, stupid, disgraceful, not deserving of love, etc. I worked hard to release all the ick in order to forgive those who did that to me. The hardest pill to swallow was realizing that none of those people did anything to me. I allowed and invited this into my life. Every single one of "those" people were simply a reflection of how I felt about myself. That was a huge shift and Ah-ha moment for me. Life was hard but worth it.

Over the past eight years I have worked to discover why I felt so terribly about myself. Why couldn't I love the person staring back at me in the mirror? Why couldn't I allow myself to receive the love others wanted to give me? The energy work I received, the classes I took and the countless healing circles I participated in brought truth to the surface and provided tools for me to make all of the discoveries I was able to explain above. I had no idea I spent my life accumulating mask after mask in order to "make it through the day." Once I discovered Reiki, I no longer wanted to simply survive, I wanted to thrive. Regular energy sessions and intuitive readings helped me keep my energy field clear of the debris that comes when processing emotions and provided the tools and guidance needed to help me continue moving forward. Classes provided me the knowledge to understand what was happening to me and

Reiki was my gateway drug to a life of spiritual service. The goal is unconditional love for myself. In my quest to reach that goal I have shed many masks and now sit here the truest, most authentic me I have ever been. Do I have all of the answers? Absolutely not. Was the work difficult? You betcha. Was it worth every effort to get to the happiness, joy, peace and love that I feel today? You'd better believe it!!

My journey is far from over. I want to share the love as it has been shared with me. I want to use my gifts to help others discover and nurture theirs. Once we have unconditional love for ourselves, we see the world and all the people in it through a different set of eyes. Collectively we can shift this world back to a place of love. Reiki provided a foundation for me to grow, evolve and transform my life. For that, I am eternally grateful. Life is...

Author Spotlight

Judy Forder

J udy is a spiritually based Energy Practitioner and Certified Intuitive Counselor. Using multiple modalities such as Reiki, Angelic Light Weaving and Axiatonal Alignment, Judy assists her clients in removing blocks which prevent them from moving forward, creating sacred space to release judgement and allow unconditional love for self and others. Using

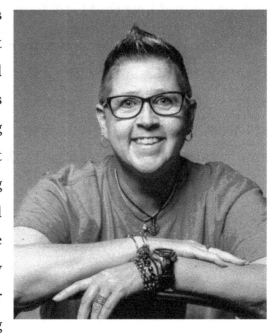

her intuition, Judy provides her clients with tools to move through the healing process and guide them on their path to reconnecting and trusting the guidance of their Soul. Judy is passionate about empowering her clients and teaches Reiki 1,2 &3/Master, Angelic Light Weaving and Axiatonal Alignment classes by request.

In December of 2012, Judy received her first Reiki session and from that day forward fully committed to releasing old outdated beliefs and emotions which were preventing her from living her best life. During her healing journey she decided she wanted to help others heal the way she was being helped by her mentors. After working to the level of Reiki Master, completing a two- year Energy Healing Course and doing healing work part time, the decision was made. In July of 2016, Judy resigned her position as a physical education teacher of 24 years to follow the guidance of her Soul and began doing her healing work full time. Judy continues to take workshops and classes to expand her knowledge and enhance her gifts. She became a Certified Intuitive Counselor in the fall of 2019.

Judy is the owner of Powered by Your Soul, LLC[1] and practices out of Journeys Holistic Health & Wellness Center of York, PA. She can be found on Facebook at Powered by Your Soul, LLC as well as Journeys with Judy and Anchors of Light. Journey with Judy is a podcast available on YouTube as well as FB and Anchors of Light is a group page where you can find live Angelic Light Weaving healing videos provided for free to all who watch.

Judy is honored to use her gifts to help you realize yours. If you are willing to do the work, no dream is too big.

---

[1] www.poweredbyyoursoul.com

Painting for My Life
Jimmy Purkey

I talk myself down from everything. It's like I'm scared to succeed, because if it falls apart – so do I.

This week I had some days off to reflect on myself, my relationship to the Divine, and my relationship with my art. Even with the meds, I'm still a bit lost in my head. When I feel that I'm not meeting my expectations, I beat myself up about it.

One day I'll love myself as much as I should.

Growing up, my grandmother taught me to be myself and to be kind. She was by far my best critic and strongest supporter. During my childhood she spoiled me through my love of reading. In my adolescence, she allowed me to be as quirky and odd as I chose because it was real and honest. Whatever medium I was creating in, she encouraged the process over product.

I am what I am in life because of the love, wisdom and guidance of my grandmother. She was the strongest woman in the world, the greatest mother and the best friend.

You'd have loved her.

I was diagnosed as Bipolar when I was sixteen. To keep myself grounded to the present when I am emotionally overwhelmed, I paint. Doesn't matter what the end result is, it's all about getting it out and grounding.

I create for the most part to break down stigma attached to mental health. It's often times easier to process, produce, and then describe certain emotional concepts through an abstraction. I enjoy creating what I do. It's very therapeutic to me and is often times the one real way for me to meditate.

One of the worst things about being a creative with mental health issues is that confidence comes infrequently if at all. Oftentimes we tend to make jokes at our own expense or undercut our abilities with broken humor. It's not funny.

When I decided to do this show at the Parliament, I knew I wanted to use my gifts to help others connect to their mental health. Getting people to write down, literally, "how does this make you feel" and post it on the wall next to the art -- when people did that in response to my creations, I knew that this was the thing I was meant to do.

I would rather paint than work. One day I'll be able to support myself through my art, but for now, my painting is work when it is healing the soul, protecting and strengthening one's inner self through meditation and reflection, and reaching out and encouraging others who are also struggling. Art of any form can be the hardest, purest work that people do, and with the greatest benefit.

Art has saved my life. I can't tell you how many times. If I can extend, then, and give back, and encourage other people to extend, to connect, and to help others, then that's my calling. That's what I'm supposed to do. Connecting to people. Connecting to my faith. Connecting to, just, everything and learning when to hold on and when to let go.

Author Spotlight
Jimmy Purkey

Jimmy Purkey is a painter from York, PA. He has led several art-based communities, such as the UpCollective, and has been a strong supporter of the Penn Street Art Bridge project and local artists who work with many different mediums.

His January show "How Does This Art Make You Feel?" at the Parliament on King Street in York encouraged visitors to express themselves directly on the wall next to the paintings.

Purkey donated a portion of the proceeds from sales during his month-long show to CHI and challenges other artists and practitioners to support community and art-based mental health projects and programs.

Jimmy Purkey can be found at:
FB: @jimmypurkeyart
IG: @jimmypurkey

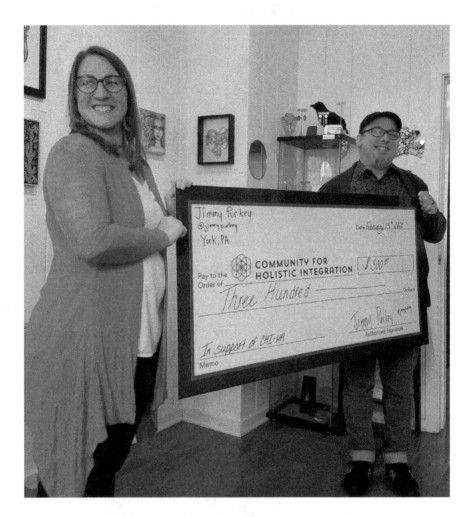

CHI Board Secretary Erin Shrader accepts Jimmy
Purkey's donation.

A Journey of Transformation
Peg Zimmerman

Transformation ... spiritual evolution ... connecting to who we really are as spirit, soul, and divine love rather than our stories...I believe that's the gift of being here on this earth, especially at this time. Almost twenty years ago, I would have "thought" I was doing and being that already, but I was about to discover differently. The beginning of my transformation began at age 47, seven years after my remarriage.

Perhaps the transformative years of women's forties and fifties are nature's way of allowing women to bring new energy and healing into their self/families at a time when most children are usually out of the home and there's more time and energy to do the seemingly intense inner healing. Hormonal issues can surface without much warning or invitation, and women typically are no longer able to suppress unresolved wounds in these years.

For me, the unresolved abandonment in my childhood reached out to "save" an abandoned and traumatized child who had lost attachment at birth and had just lost her second family. The hormonal dynamic was intensified when our daughter reached adolescence; so thus, a perfect storm was created.

Ten years later, Emotional Repatterning and other energy medicine methods integrated into psychotherapy brought transformation and greater health and freedom in our adopted child, and consequently, in me, our generational line, and beyond. It has been a process, to say the least, but I intuitively knew it was our path. I now offer not just psychotherapy, but also Emotional Repatterning (ER), muscle balancing, and many other holistic health care modalities that not just boost our immune system but also clear blockages that cause stress, disease and pain.

My roots are Christian, and I've come to understand, thanks to Caroline Myss (renowned author and speaker of human consciousness, spirituality and health), that we can't totally abandon the faith in which we are born. I have broadened my view of God, self, others and the world, though, and have integrated greater freedom of thought and being. I now believe that Divine Love is a universal, ever-present frequency and we always have that connection, source and knowledge at our avail.

Many things can get in the way of that knowing: attachment styles, dogmas, beliefs, defense mechanisms, traumas large and small. They all carry different frequencies of energy (combative, protective, emotion-based) and they all block our connectedness to our intuition, our soul knowing, and our higher frequency.

The door to alternative and holistic healthcare opened when the need was great and other options were unfruitful. The provision was so great that it was undeniable to me. Emotional repatterning and associated energy medicine techniques are powerful and effective alternatives to traditional "talk therapy" because they bypass our natural defense symptoms, which we all brilliantly and naturally develop in order to survive in our early childhood. Stored in our bodies are beliefs and thus strategies that helped us get what we needed to survive, be seen, and be loved.

The brain's natural response when our spiritual, emotional, physical, and mental needs aren't met or are threatened is fight, flight, or freeze. We all developed and have stored survival strategies. It's part of living here on this earth. Their manifestations are manifold: dependency, codependency, non-existent or limited self-care, escaping, dissociating, denial of some kind, self- or other-hate, etc. We can develop awareness and then compassion for our survival strategies, and clearing these deep-seated, limiting pain behaviors brings greater freedom and health.

ER individually reads what the body has stored and what it needs. I witnessed and experienced this transformative process and was amazed at the body's ability to always work toward homeostasis, balance and healing. I was a wife and mother to seven children, an educator, a lay counselor, a volunteer in many capacities, and a professional counselor, but now I had found my soul's delight that enhanced my other roles.

I got certified in Touch for Health (TFH), Levels I-IV, and then in, Emotional Repatterning to complement psychotherapy, as needed and desired by clients. These two forms of Applied Kinesiology can be done independently or can be integrated into psychotherapy. Both modalities use an established method of reading the balance of the body's electrical system at any given moment (muscle testing).

Connection between our heart, soul, mind, and body orchestrates deeper healing. When muscle testing is done, we are tapping into that body-mind-soul wisdom. As an integrative psychotherapist, I help clients explore the mind, body and soul connections that cause their wellness and illness, with the intention of their wholeness and well-being.

I understand that we are all energy and energy directs the healing process. My most important role is to be present in love, guidance and support as clients are active in their own healing process of honoring and respecting their journey and of coming home to the God-given knowledge of who they truly are as pure and perfect Love. Wounds happen in relationship and can only be healed in relationship. I offer a safe healing space for that to happen.

Are there places where you are not living in freedom and success due to individual issues, relational difficulty, or trauma and dis-ease? Would you value transformational coaching toward greater self-care? ER is a freeing journey of transformation. The client's intention directs the healing energy and the balancing gently and easily releases the related blocked or reactive energetic pattern of that issue. Affirmations and meridian systems are used, along with self-balancing techniques, to release stress. This non-invasive balancing is client-done by acupressure, tapping, light touch and other simple correction skills. Changes manifest on the physical, mental, emotional, biochemical and spiritual levels. ER can be done at my home office or remotely (phone, facetime, skype).

Both Muscle Balancing and ER are methods based in Touch for Health (TFH), a simple yet powerful preventative and corrective system of health care based in Applied Kinesiology (AK) and the concept of internal energy foundational in traditional Chinese medicine. The TFH training I received is based on the book *Touch for Health* by John Thie, D.C. (1973), and endorsed by the International Kinesiology College of Zurich. Arlene Green, who wrote the Emotional Repatterning method (1996) and who has strong affiliation with TFH, used techniques and information from various individuals around the world, including Dr. John Thie, Dr. Bruce Dewe and his Goal Balancing concept,

Gordon Stokes and Daniel Whiteside's One Brain system, and homeopaths Malcolm and Sue Chaffer from Sydney, Australia.

Kinesiology is the most holistic of all the natural therapies. Dr. John Thie thought kinesiology should be available not just to chiropractors but to people in all walks of life to empower them to take greater responsibility for their and their families' health and healing. Energy medicine expert and guru Donna Eden got her beginnings from TFH and then expanded it with her vibrant exercises, knowledge and personality.

Since its inception in 1970, millions of people on a global basis have benefited from TFH and the many professionally focused forms of specialized kinesiology that it's spawned. Today, in this information age, it's no secret to the average person that our body exists as both a physical and non-physical entity; that we have an energetic "blueprint" that directs the grosser manifestations of the body in its incredibly intricate workings.

Although so called primitive cultures around the world have been aware of this concept for thousands of years, our Western society has, in some ways, been a victim of its own mechanistic scientific dogma influencing modern medicine to view the body in an almost totally anatomical and physiological way. This is now rapidly changing. Perceiving the body as a multidimensional, holistic creation rather than as a complex machine makes Touch for Health an effective instrument for people to explore and harmonize these dimensions.

A fundamental premise of kinesiology is that the body has innate healing energy and is always doing its best to care for itself, but sometimes needs to be helped into a better position to achieve this care. Kinesiology is grounded in the study of anatomy and physiology and uses muscles as monitors of stress and imbalance within the body. Kinesiology recognizes the flows of energy within the body not only relate to the muscles but to every tissue and organ that make the body a living, feeling being. These energy flows can be evaluated by testing the function of the muscles, which in turn reflect the body's overall state of structural, chemical, or emotional balance. In this way, kinesiology taps into energies that the more conventional modalities overlook.

Kinesiology looks beyond symptoms and does not treat named diseases — nor does it diagnose them. Energy flow can be interrupted as the result of injury, emotional trauma, nutritional or other unresolved stress and affect the whole body. The exact nature of blockage in the energy flow can be more closely identified by muscle testing and the balancing has a flow-on effect into total body energy. Energy balancing brings a person closer to achieving any goal of their choice – in sport, relationships, learning, or coping with life generally.

Receiving a balance is ultimately about receiving validation, affirmation, and compassion. One balance does not require more balances. The process for that intention/goal is completed within the session.

Why embark on this journey for whatever length or intensity you choose? Consider that when we own our own power without self-righteousness or need for approval, we then allow others to do the same. When we have self-respect and don't limit our self, we can then respect others and more wholly contribute to society as a whole.

Author Spotlight
Peg Zimmerman

Peg Zimmerman is self-employed as an Integrative Psychotherapist with a home office in Lititz, PA. She also enjoys her work with the elderly in nursing, retirement and personal homes. Doing depression and anxiety screenings in local middle and high schools with TeenHope keeps her engaged with another segment of society that she loves.

Peg's personal and professional experience has integrated the fields of psychotherapy, education and the healing of body, mind and soul. She sees individuals in their wholeness and cooperates with them in exploring the mind-body-soul connections that affect wellness and illness, as they allow.

Peg delights in and honors her role as wife, mother to six amazing adult children and their beloved spouses, and grandma to twelve grandchildren currently. She is honored to be on this journey of life with them. Each one has been a transformational mirror to her in her own journey.

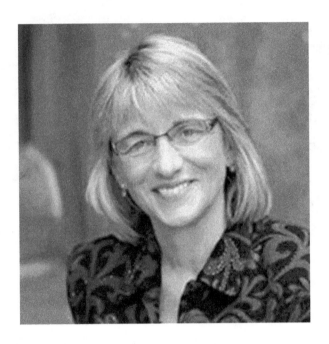

Catch up with her at

www.pegzimmerman.com

facebook.com/pegzimmermanholisticcounselor

Making Sense of the Remnants
Kimber Bowers

Pressing my mouth over his, I fought frantically to breathe life back into his limp body and I remember the initial excitement of what seemed like a gurgle of breath that quickly faded into a final exhale. There was no movement. There was no life. There was only emptiness.

And on that final exhale escaped everything I ever thought I knew... everything I ever thought I was. It felt like the very fiber of my being simply evaporated... ceased to be. My interpretation of life had been completely spun around this other being... his existence in the world and everything that I could be to him. We built dreams together and named our future children together and imagined everything that could be. I started out as a partner and became a caretaker where every choice I made was designed to support us and get us back to that dream. I had put all of myself into fighting for him. Without him, I had no idea what I was, why I was, or where I was going. I couldn't even remember where else I had ever been.

Have you ever felt that way? Have you ever suffered a loss that simply swept you off your feet? Turned the world upside down? A loss you never imagined possible to survive and yet, somehow you were confused to find yourself still existing and just couldn't make sense of what that could mean? Have you ever attached all of your purpose to a role or relationship — so much so, that without it, you didn't even understand who you were?

I lost a great love, yes, and to this day he is still missed, but it was only in grieving his loss that I discovered myself. Grief can be like that. It requires us to make sense of what remains... including ourselves and our roles in the world. For as long as I could remember, I had been defining myself through my roles and relationships, through self-proclaimed responsibilities, through what I could give, through the care I felt so called to bring. For as long as I could remember, I had made it my purpose to keep everyone else happy and safe and put my all into loving them every step of the way. For as long as I could remember, I had been waiting for someone to love me back the same way, looking for those roles to validate me. And here, when I started to think I had found it, it was ripped away.

I had identified myself through my trauma, through the things I had felt I needed that didn't seem available when I needed them, through the years of longing for a savior that never seemed to come, through the idea of myself as unlovable and the need to prove differently. I had sought to fill my own holes through the roles I played to others and I had sought to redeem myself through another's love. And it didn't always work. In fact, it seldom really went the way I planned.

I had lost friends. I had lost family. I had lost loved ones. I had lost health. I had lost abilities. I had lost plans. I had lost roles. And now, I had lost the love of my life and all of the dreams of redemption built around him in one crashing moment that seemed to shatter everything. All of the caring I did and all of the saving I had tried to do and all of the love I had given, had simply not been enough. I had failed.

I thought for sure I was supposed to be the one to save him... and maybe that's a codependent thing. He certainly wasn't the first one I had tried to save, but I had allowed this relationship to finally make sense of all the heartache I had lived up until that point. I had looked to it to validate me, my existence, and everything that I had ever doubted or regretted or allowed to make me feel like less, as all having led me to this point.

Maybe the desire to feel love sometimes gets confused as a need to prove our worthiness of love. Maybe the desire to love sometimes gets confused as a need to fix or a need to save. Maybe I felt a need to love everyone else out of a desire to believe that I myself deserved love. Maybe I just needed to believe there was goodness in the world. Maybe I needed to save everyone else in order to have hope that I, too, could one day be saved. But in reality, none of us can do any of these things for anyone but ourselves.

In the immediate space after his death, I became the failure and the guilty. I blamed myself for another non-successful rescue. I blamed myself for his death. I was still identifying myself through trauma and the shame it induced, in a new way – falling back into the self-loathing I had nearly escaped, and unable to believe I deserved to heal. The path I sought for redemption hadn't worked.

Everything in my life seemed pointless as none of it could ever prove my worth, and as a result I began to pull back and discover some space.

In that space and in that emptiness, no tomorrows planned, no dreams to fulfill, no love to save, fearful of any new connections out of an expectation to fail again, I began to really look for meaning inside myself. In the void left behind, I had to figure out who I really was and what I wanted to bring on my own. These were questions I had never asked myself and none of them were easy. I had never allowed myself to fully grieve any losses of the past. Instead, I had merely shouldered the shame and thrown myself into the next role or relationship, struggling to meet the perceived expectation that would somehow make me worthy. I was always too busy trying to appease everyone else, trying to earn that validation.

It became increasingly apparent that every single choice I had ever made in my life was made out of the perceived need to secure love... to be seen as enough... to undo the aftermath of childhood trauma that told me I wasn't.

There was a part of me that always sensed a larger connection, but I hadn't seen much evidence of it in my life. There was a part of me that had always believed love must be available, I just hadn't figured out how to let it flow into my life. There was a part of me that knew I was enough, but there were too many mental barriers preventing me from accepting that in my life.

In the stillness, I was guided to journey within and consciously process the traumas and relationships of my past through a series of cognitive questions and in doing so, I was finally able to move forward with intention. I was finally able to discover a deeper identity and I was finally able to believe I deserved something good in my life, a process which today I guide others through in my work as a Spiritual Counselor and Clinical Hypnotherapist. I was finally able to get my brain on board with my soul. I was finally able to release the need for validation... to put down the shame and to recognize that I was enough already, just as I was.

Things started to shift and new opportunities presented themselves. I began to understand all the negative interpretations that began in my own brain. I began to understand how to build my own positive evidence so that I could break through them to feel more supported and more deserving.

Through a combination of conscious processing, energy work, and hypnotherapy, I was able to reconnect myself to that inner knowing mentally, emotionally, and spiritually. I was able to build new neural pathways and create healthier thought patterns. I was able to build my self-trust and spiritual connection and start stepping through them in the world.

After decades of relentlessly judging myself for all my failures to everyone else and feeling trapped in the misaligned life I'd created, I accepted myself as the long-awaited savior. I went from feeling trapped in endless expectations to feeling free to be me, and actually understanding who that is. I went from a desperate need to be loved to a deep inner knowing that I am love and have the ability to give myself love right here and right now. Allowing that flow of love into my life has completely changed my experience.

There is joy in the knowing and in the expression. There is fulfillment in recognizing the enoughness that you bring into each step of this ongoing journey. There is resilience in knowing that enoughness regardless of the outcome. After years of interpreting everything as further evidence against myself, I have found the freedom to see the beauty of all that I am in connection to Spirit, and step into a fuller expression.

I get it. There are so many losses and there are so many remnants... and there are so many pieces of things that maybe we think we are or are supposed to be... and sometimes the idea of doing anything with them is simply overwhelming. Everything happens for a reason. Everything propels something in some manner or form. The pieces you have are exactly what is needed to grow forward. By assembling the remnants of our experience in a way that supports us right now, by acknowledging that we deserve to have that support on our growth journey, everything can change.

If you are struggling with the remnants, sitting in a pile of pieces from the things you've lost, with no idea of how to find peace with where you are — it begins by recognizing that you have a choice. You can stay in the brokenness, or you can begin to put whatever pieces you have together as best you can, assuming that everything you have is here to support you in some way. You can ask, "How do I grow through this?" And you can allow yourself to do just that, to put it all together in way that supports your growth and expression right now. You get to decide how the pieces fit. It isn't always easy, and I get that. It is, however, *possible.*

If you find yourself struggling, there is support. There are pages of people here who have made similar journeys and are devoted to sharing their wisdom. Explore them. Each of us has a light within us that the world needs, and I think I am speaking on behalf of all CHI's holistic practitioners when I say, it is our goal to unleash as many stars as possible! Are you ready to shine?

Worksheet: Pieces of Me

I am passionate about:	I find joy:
_____	_____
_____	_____
_____	_____

I find meaning in:	My top values are:
_____	_____
_____	_____

My top interests are:	The gifts I bring include:
_____	_____
_____	_____

The "why" behind my being:
_____
_____
_____

Use this chart to identify some of the pieces you have. Recognize anywhere that they may overlap in the "why" behind your being. Decide how to honor these pieces in your life.

Author Spotlight

Kimber Bowers

Rev. Kimber Bowers CCHt is an Amazon Bestselling Author, mom, artist, and Integrative Mind Body Wellness Practitioner holding a degree in Transpersonal Mind-Body Psychology and certifications in Coaching, Reiki, Clinical Hypnotherapy, & Spiritual Counseling.

As an empath who suffered most of her life with PTSD, Clinical Depression, and Anxiety, she has now discovered the keys to joy and fulfillment and has made it her mission to help you find yours!

Her personal twenty years' experience of trauma and depression in combination with over a decade of spiritual and psychological study give her a unique understanding of those whom she serves.

It is her goal to serve as a reflection of the love that IS so that others can discover it within their own hearts and within their own lives.

Her group program, *Open & Receive: 4 Steps to Unleash Fulfillment,* guides women to release the traumas of the past and establish a secure identity allowing them to move forward with sustainable purpose & fulfilment now. www.lovinglighthw.com/open-receive

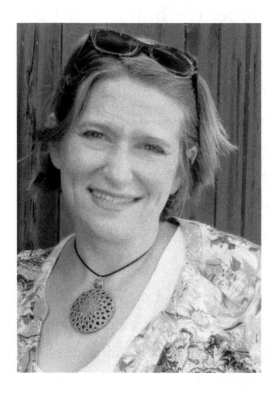

Kimber Bowers

Loving Light Holistic Wellness 410-241-2635

www.lovinglighthw.com

Find it on Facebook

Check out her books at bit.ly/KimberBowers

Coming Back to Life
The Rebel Herbalist, Erin Shrader

I stand in the icy rain, listening as the tiny pebbles of ice hit the snow. The full wolf moon illuminates the clouds even as they blanket her. The cedars lean their wizard capped tops toward the earth, growing heavy with the burden of winter's snow and ice. I can feel their wisdom, their ancient memories, their rootedness in the ways of the ancestors.

I call out to this land on which I make my home and raise my family; whose living water I drink from deep within our well, whose wood I burn in our stove to warm our family, whose medicine I collect and dry and tincture and blend into salve, whose berries and nuts and leaves I collect to eat and feed my family. I ask this land whose water runs in my veins to give me wisdom to speak with you. I ask this land to show me how to tend the well.

"Teach me how to live in harmony with you. My people have forgotten. We cannot remember how to live in a way that honors all of life. Please speak to me and I will use my gifts to speak your message into the world of humans as best I can." I plead with the spirits of this land,

and my heart overflows with love and longing for a future that honors all of life.

This land has been reluctant to accept my love. It is wounded and mistrustful of humans. I could feel a cold icy glare from deep in the forest for the first few months that we lived here. One day as I walked in the forest, I approached an old tree whose roots were growing in a twisted bridge across the small stream that divides the land between our home and the neighbor's property.

This tree is an old oak tree with four sturdy trunks that all grew up from the same root ball. The tree was surrounded by heavily armored raspberry bushes and poison ivy[2]. I could feel that this tree was heavily guarded and not easily accessible.

In my haste to deeply connect to the spirit of this land, I pushed my way through the plant guardians and approached this giant. I was looking for a powerful spot where I could visit every day to commune with the land and watch the seasons pass. I asked the tree permission to visit every day and cultivate a relationship. I had carried a green jasper stone in my pocket and placed it deep into a scar in the tree bark. I had asked the stone to carry my intention as a vibration, to help the tree to understand my request.

---

[2] My healer friend calls poison ivy "Sister Protectress."

Even as I placed the stone and offered my intention to the oak, the wind began to pick up. Suddenly, the sky was thick with grey clouds where there had just been blue skies. The grove of maple trees nearby were rubbing their branches together in the gathering wind, making loud groaning sounds. The breeze turned cold. My skin prickled in goosebumps. I was not wanted here. I could feel it in my bones. I was being warned by the spirit of the land itself. Leave. Now.

I walked back to the house in a disoriented fog. I had been very energetically affected by my experience in the forest. I felt confused, foggy-brained, unsure of my footing. I pulled myself back together and had some chocolate to help me get grounded back into my body.

The next day I gathered my courage to go back to the forest to get an answer from the old oak tree. I went to the place where I had left the intention stone and reached inside the deep pocket where I had placed the stone. It wasn't there. It was impossible for this stone to have fallen out of this pocket. It was a doughnut shaped hole in the bark, a scar from an injury long ago. The center well was deep and gravity would have had no power to pull the stone from this pocket. And yet, the stone was missing.

I kneeled down and looked in the thick briars at the base of the tree. There I found my jasper stone. The message was clear. The stone was rejected. I was not wanted here. I paid my respects to the tree, offered my gratitude for the powerful work it is doing on this land, and made my way to the grove of maples that had groaned and waved and called to me the day before.

Here among the maples, I found a large white quartz, completely above the ground. This stone was approximately the size of a microwave. I sat upon the stone and reflected on my interaction with the oak. I know that the land here is stressed. We are plagued with the ash borer beetle and the cedar rust fungus, as well as overly wet clay soil. The mountain above our home has been deforested for agriculture, and this valley we live in has taken on much more rain runoff than it has ever experienced before. The earth here is taxed, and I sense that its energy is being used in healing and holding its ground. We only have one surviving adult ash tree on the property, and many dead skeletons from the borer beetle. We have lost five cedar trees just this year. The locusts are dying from a combination of the beetles and the wetness. Most of the new saplings I have planted have died.

As I sat feeling the heaviness of this struggle for the land to accommodate the burden of human activity, my eyes were drawn to the area around me. Here, on this quartz slab, in the shade of a grove of mature, healthy maple trees, I found myself in a nursery. All around me were young ash trees. There were hundreds of them, anywhere from yearlings to five-year-old saplings. The forest is regenerating. Life continues. Maybe one of these saplings will have the genetic profile that resists the borer. My heart filled with hope. I had found my sacred place on this land after all.

In her book *Garden Awakening,* Mary Reynolds explores the deep consciousness of the land itself. She offers tools and advice about how to work with this consciousness as we remember how to steward and partner with the land that we live on and with. By connecting to and listening to the land, its creatures, its waters and winds, we are able to make decisions about how we interact with and change the topography in ways that are respectful and healthy to the land itself. This way of belonging to the land with sacred intention and learning to take the time to truly listen is not a foreign concept. Cultures who are immersed in nature continue to listen carefully to the land, even today. They know that to do so preserves their health as much as it protects the life of the land.

We have become powerful beyond measure as individuals, and we have collectively become a force that shapes life on Earth. This era of history has been called the Anthropocene[3] as a way to designate the formative/

---

[3] From "anthropos," the Greek word for human

destructive effects of the human species. Our collective activities have changed the climate and the landscape on Earth. From clear-cut mining operations to agro-business, and from the construction of cities and sprawling suburbs, we have carved and sculpted and formed the landscape with our giant machines. In our efforts to make life comfortable and profitable (for a few) we have toppled the dominos in a cascading effect of large-scale destruction. Scientists warn that we are living within a major extinction event, with over half of the world's land and sea creatures expected to be extinct by the year 2100[4]. This extinction event lies firmly on the shoulders of human activity.

How did we get here?

Paul Levy, in his book *Dispelling Wetiko,* describes the mind virus that has shaped the destructive force behind human activities. Native Americans had been aware of this tendency of the human toward greed and accumulation, finding its ultimate pathogenic expression in the phenomenon of the cannibal. They had been tracking this violent tendency for thousands of years and had found ways of addressing it within their own cultures. They called this sickness Wetiko in the Cree language[5]. The Native Americans believed that nearly all of the European colonists

---

[4] www.nationalgeographic.com/science/prehistoric-world/mass-extinction/
[5] windigo in Ojibway, wintiko in Powhatan

were infected with this mind virus, and that it is highly contagious.

This disconnection from the web of life and focus on aggrandizing the self is the hallmark of the empire building western cultures of the world. For several thousand years, a small group of powerful men have been riding the wave of power that some unknown force unleashed on the world. Perhaps this force is an evil being (like the Christian Satan or the Buddhist Mara) or perhaps this force is the shadow aspect of power in the collective human psyche that has run rampant, hitched to the belief that progress for its own sake is valuable. I don't think that we can know exactly how we collectively fell prey to this system of belief, but I do believe that it is time for us to take a clear-eyed look at the world that we have participated in creating

By collectively agreeing that the planet is inert, not alive, simply a collection of resources for humans to use and dominate, we have severed the thread that connects humans to the larger web of life. We no longer see ourselves in the majesty of the sunrise, recognize our own innocence in the wide eyes of the doe, or our own cleverness in the fox's late night maneuvers around the chicken house. We no longer see the purity of our tears in the running stream or our boundless passion as the thunderclouds roll in from the southwest. Our ancestors knew that the natural world was the first scripture, and that all human musings have been only an attempt to understand what nature holds as pure and sacred truth.

Living a life that is divorced from the world around us has left us abandoned. We are craving belonging and connection, but we're projecting our sense of betrayal as a way of coping with our wounds. The need for border walls, for more and more assurances of safety from the frightening "other" is a symptom of our infection with the Wetiko mind virus. We are obsessed with our own safety, our own fortune, amassing our own wealth. And in our obsession, everyone who is different than us is a potential threat to our safety. We are terrified because we know that we do not belong here. We do not belong in this world that we have created. Our animal bodies are gripped with fear. We are overwhelmed, overstimulated, undernourished. We crave the nourishment of minerals and healthy fats. We crave the nourishment of touch. We crave the nourishment of stories and wisdom and laughter. We crave leisure and deep rest and slow time. We are starving.

In her book, *Belonging,* Toko-pa Turner offers us a solution to our sense of fragmentation and soul-level starvation. She posits that belonging is actually a set of skills over which we can gain competency. As humans, we have evolved to learn how to belong based on social cues and norms within societies, just as we learn to walk and speak. In our current culture, we are not provided a framework for the development of strong social bonds and so we do not develop the skill set for belonging. We don't learn how to belong to the Earth, how to belong to ourselves, how to belong to the Sacred Mystery, how to belong to our families, our communities, the larger world or the cosmos. We have inflated the individual self so much and put so much emphasis on the success of the self, that even our religions and New Age spiritualities have lost the art of connection in the race to the pinnacle of personal perfection.

Toko-pa suggests several skills that we can develop in the art of belonging. She describes learning how to hand-make items like baskets and food and other forms of art and everyday practical tools. She talks about creating what she calls beauty medicine, being able to create something beautiful wherever you find yourself.

Maybe you leave a cairn at the side of the road on your evening walk, a piece of enchantment for a neighbor to find later. Maybe you weave daisy chains and leave them hanging from trees. There is a movement in my local area where people paint stones and leave them in random places for other people to find. These small acts of kindness and beauty weave us into the larger life of our community.

My son and I found one of these painted stones while we were walking a trail in the state forest. It was so enchanting to him, and now he has begun to look more attentively for magic everywhere we go. In his looking, he is seeing more of the world around us. In his deep seeing of the world, he is belonging himself to it. He is seeing where the moon rises, finding that tiny hummingbird nest, seeing how the bark peels from the cedar trees and the river birch. The world is full of stories and mysteries and magic for us to experience.

I am privileged to serve on the board of directors for the Horn Farm Center for Agricultural Education[6] in Hellam, PA. At the Horn Farm, we use regenerative agricultural practices and permaculture practices to listen deeply to the land as we make decisions in partnership with the soil, the plants, the trees and insects. By working with the staff at the Horn Farm, I have learned that the health of food plants is promoted and protected by the health of the ecosystem surrounding the farm fields.

The health of the forests improves water quality and habitat for beneficial predators (the kind of predators that eat insects, rabbits and groundhogs that would like to eat crop plants). The health of the streams and forests checks runoff from massive rainfall, preserving nutrient rich topsoil for growing optimally nutritious food. Working with perennial crops and agroforestry requires less resources

---

[6] www.hornfarmcenter.org

and improves yields. There are so many ways that we can work in a wiser, more conscious way with the world around us. As Gerard Manley Hopkins tries to illuminate in his poem, *As Kingfishers Catch Fire*[7], all of nature is communicating itself to us all of the time. Nature tells us who it is, what it needs, and how to participate mindfully in the amazing dance that unfolds all around us.

The plants themselves hold a very real and tangible consciousness. I have never experienced more miracles than when working consciously with the plants.

A few years ago, I had purchased some very high-quality motherwort seeds from a reputable dealer. I planted the seeds and watered them all spring, but never saw them sprout. Saddened, I gave up the idea of having motherwort in my garden and bought a tincture instead.

Two years later, I became pregnant with our son. While working in the garden I noted a large and prolific weed taking over one of the beds. I couldn't believe it, but this "weed" was motherwort. She was growing very near to where I had planted the seeds two years before. The tincture I made from this spontaneous growth of motherwort in my garden was instrumental in inducing my labor and calming my postpartum nervousness, as well as helping me heal from some significant birth trauma. I firmly believe that

---

[7] https://www.poetryfoundation.org/poems/44389/as-kingfishers-catch-fire

those seeds laid dormant in the soil until I needed their medicine the most.

Last summer I had become fascinated with mugwort, a plant associated with Artemis, the moon and the power of dreaming. I had been doing intense dreamwork while studying Toko-pa Turner's book, and I was hoping to connect with mugwort to help me in my dreaming. I started asking friends if they knew where a stand of mugwort was growing so that I could harvest some for my dreamwork. All of my leads were coming up short and I was starting to give up on finding mugwort in my area.

One afternoon, after dropping our daughter off at a friend's house, I got a very strong urge to drive the two hours to my brother's house near Philadelphia. My husband, who has grown used to these types of thing, was agreeable and we made the trip very spontaneously. Shortly after arriving, I discovered a small mugwort plant growing directly in the middle of my brother's stone driveway! I nearly fainted! We transplanted the mugwort successfully, and she has been a powerful ally in my dreaming, and in so many other ways as well.

After a very satisfying visit to the annual Horn Farm Center plant sale last spring I came home the very proud mother of a baby tulsi plant (holy basil). I had been looking forward to connecting with Tulsi[8] for a while, and I was so excited to bring the plant into my garden.

When I began to prepare the soil for transplanting Tulsi, it became clear that she wasn't to be planted in the garden. I could feel a strong "no" emanating from the plant. There is a way to feel yes/no easily within the body. My healer friend Jen[9] taught me about the Ping/Thud method. When the body is feeling a "yes" it feels like a high-pitched ping within the heart center, almost propelling my body forward. When the body is feeling "no" it feels like a dull thud or a dropping sensation in the belly. I was feeling a very clear thud when trying to plant Tulsi in the garden. I took a step back, deepened my breath and looked up at the sky. I saw a clear image in my mind of a potted plant. Tulsi wanted to be potted. And she wanted to be close to the house.

From that moment, Tulsi spent the summer in a lovely pot by the front door of our home. She grew so big and robust in that pot that she began to topple over from the weight of her branches, heavy with flowers and always full of bumble bees and pollinator flies. Late last fall I received a new book called The Illustrated Herbiary. In this book it describes the Indian custom of keeping tulsi by the

---

[8] Like rose and lily, tulsi is normally not capitalized. In this article however, Tulsi is capitalized when the plant and the author are invested in a relationship.
[9] Brigidsway.com

front door of the home. Her enchanting scent is said to remind all who pass by about their own sacredness, and to act as a bridge between heaven and earth. By listening to her, I was able to allow her to more fully express her gifts.

Cultivating a relationship with the plants, the land around us, the living waters, the feathered and scaled ones, our own wild hearts, this is the antidote to Wetiko. Finding ourselves in love with the world, seeing all of Life as our kin, remembering how to steward the flow of energy through its cycles of life and death, this is the rightful place of the power of the human.

In my work as an herbalist, I often say that I am bringing people back to life. What I mean by that is my work reconnects humans to the web of life. We don't "take an herb" to alleviate a troublesome symptom. We encounter a plant and enter into a sacred relationship where the plant is the teacher, the guide, and the healer. Our relationship with these plant allies not only heals our symptoms, it reconnects us to our wild hearts, our deeply intuitive minds, and our radiant souls.

Won't you come back to life?

Author Spotlight

Erin Shrader

Erin Shrader, RN, BSN, RYT is an herbalist tending the Sacred Grove in Dover, PA. She is trained as a Registered Nurse, Yoga Teacher, Spiritual Director, Reiki Master and Herbalist. She serves as CHI Board Secretary. Erin has been seeking Divine in nature and searching for ways to end suffering for as long as she can remember.

Connect with Erin at therebelherbalist.com or therebelherbalit@gmail.com

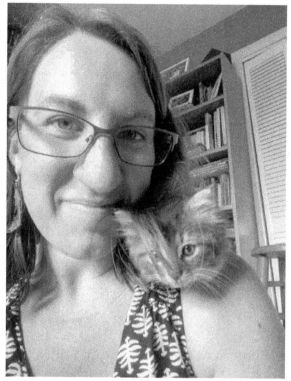

Erin Shrader, The Rebel Herbalist

What Makes Your Heart Sing?
Linda Felch

The Wixarika are an indigenous group living in the Sierra Madre mountains of Mexico. They are known for being one of the few indigenous groups that have maintained their pre-Columbian traditions, practicing their shamanic ritual and healing work for many hundreds of years. The Wixarika celebrate a continuous cycle of rituals, pilgrimages and devotional practices in their life to help them stay connected to their ancestral ways and the various gods that exist as living presences in their daily experience.

In the Wixarika tradition, the training of a shamanic healer begins by a calling through dreams and other experiences, which after being verified by the elders of the tradition, is followed by a rigorous apprenticeship involving pilgrimages to sacred sites, receiving instructions and intensive personal change. This culminates in the apprentice's initiation into the tradition. At that time the apprentice receives the title of *mara'akame,* or traditional healer, and is authorized and encouraged to begin their practice of healing.

My work as a mara'akame seeks to restore balance in the lives of my clients and connection with the energies of the sacred, living world around us. One does not need to have a manifested physical illness to benefit from this work.

This is the story of Ann, who came to me with concerns about her life purpose and her work in the world at this time in her life. A few years previously she had retired from a position in government and began searching for a path to new work that was more fulfilling.

She had trained in an alternative healing modality and developed a small healing practice.

As we sat before the Fire, Ann spoke of her involvement in her spiritual path and thoughts about getting more involved in that. She talked about how much she enjoyed her healing practice. She had recently attended a few births as a doula (something she had trained in long ago), and was considering midwifery school, with the intention of bringing her healing work to help in the birthing process.

As I did a limpia on her, cleaning away obstacles and bringing blessings into her life, I felt called to work on the area of her womb. As the two of us talked after the treatment, we speculated on what she might be ready to bring forth, to give birth to, in her own life. I encouraged her to stay open and see what showed up for her, rather than drawing conclusions right away. I left her with a question to hold open in her life: "What makes your heart sing?"

When next I saw her for a treatment, she had been researching midwifery schools and found an intensive one-year program that she liked. And something new was showing up in her life: she was being asked to take a part-time position at the place she had done her healer training. She was excited about both possibilities but didn't feel that she could do both. She decided to take care of pre-requisites for midwifery school while committing to six months at the other position.

Recently, I saw Ann again. She had let go of the idea of going back to school and was immersed in her new position. Her new job is all about shepherding her healing modality, which is not well-known, into the world. She is working to build awareness of that medicine, supporting the healers who are already out in the world, and is helping to reorganize the training. As a woman past her child-bearing years, Ann is helping to give birth to something that is important in this world and important to her. Her life has purpose and meaning and is fulfilling to her.

It fascinates me that so often the world brings us exactly what we need, so long as we are open to receiving it. Too often, our minds get stuck on a particular idea, and on making that thing happen. When we leave the door open for the world to show us what it wants from us, we can find ourselves doing things that make our hearts sing in ways we could not have imagined.

I find this to be true in my own life. My life is so much better in so many ways than I could ever have imagined when I began this journey twenty years ago.

Author Spotlight
Linda Felch

L inda is initiated as a Mara'akame in the tradition of the Wixarika (Huichol) people of Mexico. She is part of the Groupo de Tatewari (Grandfather Fire's Group), who are Westerners initiated as mara'akate (traditional healers) in the Wixarika tradition. As people who grew up in our Western culture, these healers are uniquely qualified to bring this important and powerful traditional medicine to our people, with a deeply felt and lived knowledge of the disconnection and dis-ease of those living in our culture at this time.

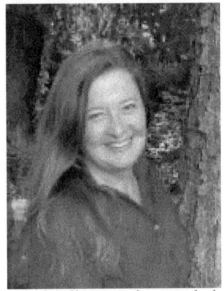

Linda offers deep shamanic healing sessions to help you move through the stuck places in your life, to heal on all levels, and to support you in becoming more fully who you are meant to be in this life.

As in most indigenous traditions, Wixarika healing works with the root spiritual cause of illness, seeking to restore balance in our lives and connection with the energies of the sacred world. **Find her on Facebook or at** healingwithnature.org

A Fresh Approach to Personal Change
Pattie Craumer

"Mindfulness made easy."
"Digital coaching in 3 minutes a day."
"Brighter, smarter, happier. "
"Fast and enduring results."

Positive Prime is a fresh new approach to personal change. With thousands of topics from world class experts, it's comparable to a vision board brought to life.

Would you like to be healthier and happier while performing at a higher level, with greater ease and less anxiety? Are you someone who resists change? Asking yourself these questions usually means a silent nod. But what if you could shift your thoughts around change so it became easy, comfortable, and fun? And what if there was a simple tool to help you move through the changes you desire in ten minutes (or less) a day?

Maybe you'd like a 35-year-old body in your 50-year-old self. Or a new job that aligns with your passions. Maybe you've been dreaming of a new adventure that scares the heck out of you! Whatever your fear or anxiety around change, it's virtually universal that we humans resist change. Why?

We are creatures of habit and our brains are wired that way. Whatever we do is reflected in circuits of neurons in our brains. The neurons wire together and expand as we repeat thoughts, behaviors, and actions over time. So, the more we do something, the stronger these circuits become. That's fine if we like that habit and it supports who we are and what we want in life. But if not, ouch!

Although humans are creatures of habit, we are also inherently created for change, because we've had to stay nimble across thousands of years just to survive. And it has been discovered that our brains are plastic, or malleable, which means they can change. This is a particularly hopeful sign for the change averse person. We can alter our mindset to make change and all sorts of habits that rule our lives much easier. Using Positive Prime, it's possible to bring anything new into your life that you want, without serious effort.

I use Positive Prime every day. It's kind of like brushing my teeth. I wouldn't want to do without it. I've seen transformations in my life around being happier in the midst of strife, gaining sales confidence and managing my life as a caregiver for my father when I felt like I was falling apart.

As a caregiver, I went from feeling alone in my plight and overwhelmed with new responsibilities for my Dad's health and wellbeing, to carrying a sense of control and empowerment around being the best daughter I could. In addition, I felt much less alone and lost in my role. This was due to comforting and relevant images and statements in the Caring for the Caregiver session that I saw every day. My mind started to believe that I could handle it all and that I had company on the journey.

I have specifically used the Super Sales session to calm my nerves before a presentation. It has also helped me to change my mindset around sales, where I have felt lacking in confidence more than once in my life. Instead of feeling anxious and inadequate, after I watch this session, I'm confident, with a positive attitude towards my conversations.

I have helped others transform around food phobias and blocks around exercise. For example, my friend Kim (the creator of Positive Prime) despised walnuts. One day, after months of watching Positive Prime sessions around healthy eating, she found herself reaching for a walnut. Catching herself and enjoying the taste, she asked herself how that could be. And then she remembered Positive Prime sessions with walnuts! Her appetite for walnuts had changed.

At the corporate level, big things also can happen when employees make Positive Prime a daily habit. One multinational company in Australia ran a test on the potential impact of Positive Prime with their travel agents in training. Thirty people watched Positive Prime three times a day throughout their course. At the end of the course, the entire group not only scored better than all previous classes had, but they also didn't cram the night before and were confident and stress free as they took the final test.

Most of us rely on willpower and motivation to break a habit, face a daunting change, or abandon a limiting belief. And it's been said that to institute a new habit takes sixty-six days, so willpower and massive desire are musts. Who will stick with something that takes that long? Some will, most won't.

Technology today means that I can simply speak out loud and change my lights or my thermostat in my smart home. And I can simply use the Positive Prime tool on my computer or phone to change my mindset to become better, brighter, healthier, or even learn something new. Through a series of a thousand images and slides that move across my computer or phone like a dynamic, personalized vision board, my conscious and subconscious mind is flooded.

Each image is carefully chosen for its neuro-scientific value. Images of awe, for example, make people feel good, feel wonder, and feel a rush of positive emotions like joy and gratitude. The response to awe is linked to greater health and wellbeing. It also sparks critical thinking in the brain.

People using Positive Prime see smiles, but not just any kind of smiles. These are Duchenne smiles, notably called for their sincerity and pure radiance in the face, which uplift people and keep their minds open to messages around change.

What else is special about a Positive Prime session? People may speed up or slow down every session -- slower if they want to read each affirmation and process each image and statement in their conscious mind, and faster if they want to bypass their conscious critical judgment pre-frontal cortex, and let their other than conscious mind, the non- judgment center, absorb what you see. This second part of the brain is where habits and limiting beliefs live and hold on tight, to keep people feeling safe and comfortable...even if those habits and limits don't serve the person anymore!

Positive Prime also encourages personalization of every session with a person's own pictures, music, and favorite statements or quotes. When people see themselves in sessions, their minds align with past successes and memories, reinforcing the positives. If people have been holding negative thoughts around something in their lives, seeing these highly personalized snapshots of family, life, milestones, dreams, etc. not only enriches their enjoyment of each session but also is even more engaging.

Positive Prime is an ideal way to feature businesses, brands, or unique messages for clientele. Users can build team camaraderie, introduce new employees to new corporate values and missions. Users can teach new concepts and ideas in dynamic, customized, corporate sessions. Please dream generously, as this little tool is quite the powerhouse for the mind. Positive Prime, in a nutshell, helps brains shift into a positive state to make any desired change easier and lasting.

When looking at behaviors and changes, how do you see yourself making progress? For me, Positive Prime has delivered. I have watched sessions like Money Keys to get me unstuck from my limiting beliefs around money and abundance. And I have consistently relied on Achieving Goals to keep me focused when I wanted to rely on excuses to not deliver on my goals instead! Maybe my next Positive Prime sessions will be on manifesting the man of my dreams. Whatever I choose from the growing online library, I love having a 'go-to' tool to help me live more positively, with ease and joy, and lead others do the same.

For more information or to choose your first FREE Positive Prime session, please contact Pattie Craumer.

Author Spotlight
Pattie Craumer

Pattie has nearly 30 years' experience as an educator, speaker, and coach, connecting with audiences and individuals locally and globally. She has helped entrepreneurs solve business challenges and families adopt healthy, toxin free lifestyles, as well as coached hundreds through life's obstacles. She is a leading, certified Positive Prime Professional and Life Mastery and Dream Builder consultant. Pattie is an optimist, change agent, researcher, and problem solver who figures things out with others. She is committed to helping people to access their inherent power and potential and then deliver it into the world.

For your first FREE session with Positive Prime, go to https://app.positiveprime.com/signup.

Use Referral Code: joyful

As you share with others, future sessions are yours for free!

To personalize your session, please contact Pattie for details.

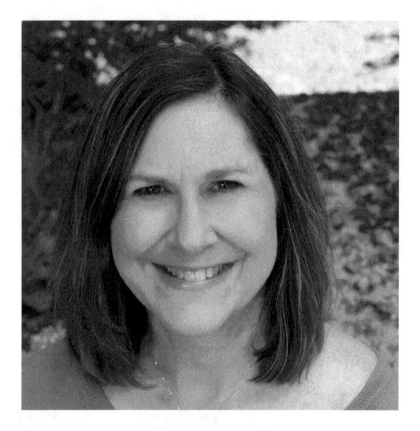

Pattie Craumer, Making Possibilities Real
Cell: (717) 421-1229
Email: pattiec7@gmail.com
Instagram: pattie_craumer
Facebook: groups/makingpossibilitiesreal/

Therapeutic Art
Louise Kemper

I am a Reiki Master, an Artist, a CHI Ambassador and co-owner of The Center of Balance LLC. located in Greencastle, Pennsylvania. As a CHI Ambassador, it is important to think outside of the box of what is considered the norm of holistic modalities. Some might not think of art as a holistic modality but when art is used in different ways it can and does provide a healing quality. Art can help one by allowing insight which can lead to self-awareness and self-healing. Art can be used as a tool for meditation or in the practice of mindfulness. Holistic treatment to me is about treating the whole person, where the mental, social, and physical are all intimately interconnected. I know first-hand the power of art as a self-healing treatment from a holistic perspective.

During a major challenge in my life, I sought mainstream counseling treatments. During counseling, I was matched with four different counselors. With the first three, it was always a bit of a challenge. It is like starting anew each time, having to retell and relive everything all over again. The fourth counselor I was matched with was an Art Therapist. Despite being an Artist, I did not consider art as having a potential place in a counseling environment and was even skeptical on how art could help me with my healing.

I will share a few personal examples of how art can be used to make a difference or change one's perspective of self. Art can be and is very instrumental in the practice of mindfulness. Mindfulness is also a form of meditation that resonates at the very core of the self. It is the purposed intent of focusing on an exact moment or specific activity. Mindfulness allows one to shut out the negatives, the busyness, the noise and to just focus on the pure moment of being or doing. An example of mindful art is when working with your hands, such as working with clay. Whether we are manually working a piece of clay to create a sculpture or something as simple as a pinch-pot or we are spinning clay on a wheel (known as throwing) to create a vessel, we are fully focused and intent on the activity as we are completing it.

Another example of how art can provide healing is from experiences of art at the tactile level. This is art that is created, can be touched and can be felt. Some say that tactile art is at the level of communication. When we are creating tactile art, we are communicating with and through our soul. When we use tactile art in a therapeutic environment, it can speak into our core and provide insight into ourselves. Tactile art has a main purpose to help create an environment for people to feel and to "see" something at an emotional level. Tactile art can also be very successful helping persons with blindness be able to see and have vision to comprehend what they are feeling or seeing.

A final example of therapeutic art is to create art and use that art as a mirror, which allows one to see what they might be feeling and provide a reflection of sorts. It can be used to allow for visual awareness of self-interpretations. For example, in my treatment I was asked to sketch an inanimate object that I felt represented how I felt about myself at the very point in my life that I was at. I drew a picture of a vase because I was in my transition to my spiritual and holistic self, so the vase represented that I was a container that could hold all of the gifts I felt that I was receiving in my journey. But I also drew a large crack in the vase, because I had the perception that the vase could not really keep things inside because there was a crack. Seeing it on paper allowed me to recognize that I felt that I was damaged and broken. It allowed me to self-interrelate that while I felt like an open vessel ready to hold things, I was not able to hold my light because of how I felt about myself, broken and not usable.

Other sketches allowed me to recognize that I took ownership of things that were negative and not really mine to own. For example, I had to draw a facial portrait of myself with my non-dominant hand, which surprisingly looked like me. However, subtle things within my sketch provided much insight into who I am, how I think and feel, and of what I have taken ownership. Not drawing parts have meanings based on the context of the picture. For example, not drawing my ears meant that I could not hear or chose not to hear my internal dialogue within my soul as related to my challenges.

Using the therapies of art has allowed me to see myself and has provided me with insight about who I am and how I thought at that point in my life. I was thankfully mistaken. We now try to incorporate therapeutic flavors of all types of art within various holistic treatments. We recognize and practice the art of drumming, music, poetry, sketching, painting, jewelry making, clay, abstracts, journaling, dancing, gardening, a physical connection to Mother Earth. The list can go on and on.

Finally, regardless of whether you perceive yourself to not have a lick of talent or you are a bona fide artist, embrace art and the gifts that art can bring into your life by enriching you and allowing you to grow in how you perceive yourself.

Author Spotlight
Louise Kemper

Local Pennsylvania born artist Louise Kemper works in many mediums; glass fusing, acrylics, abstract arts, pen and inks, pencils, watercolors, throwing clay, metals, jewelry-making, and much more. Louise likes to mix mediums up and play around with her art, using every day and odd items in her work. Louise is self-taught in many of the mediums she works in and she has been teaching classes in those mediums for more than thirty-five years. For her, art provides a means to center, balance, and rejuvenate one's self. Louise believes art is therapeutic in nature and strives to bring awareness to others as to the gift of art that is hidden within all of us. She has taught both young children and adults of all ages. Her work has also been shown and sold in New Mexico, Pennsylvania, West Virginia, Mississippi, and Maryland. Louise has won many awards for her unique, one of a kind, glass-fused jewelry, sculptures and other specialty art items. She has incorporated her art into her holistic journey.

https://thecenterofbalancellc.com/contact

Louise is co-owner of a holistic wellness center with her twin sister Leslie Punt. The Center of Balance, LLC, located at 29 N Jefferson Street, in Greencastle, PA 17225, was established officially on March 1, 2018. Louise is a Reiki Master/Wellness

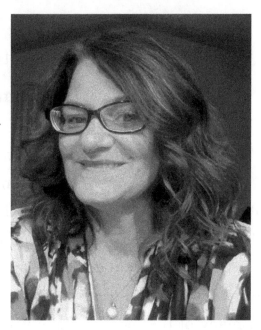

Instructor/Artist/Young Living Oil Representative. Louise's sister Leslie is a Reflexologist/ Reiki Master/ Consulting Hypnotist/ Esthetics Skincare Consultant and Holistic Health Practitioner.

Offerings at The Center of Balance include healing modalities of Reiki, Foot/Body Reflexology, Hypnosis, Massage, Skincare Consulting, holistic instructions, arts and classes, and a unique artisan gift shop.

Select Poems
Laile Wilson

Strong Women

Trying to understand
Why the voices of strong women
Have died?
Crying tears of sorrows
Pains
Carrying .
Birthing
Motherhood
Wife?

With no-name games*,
Men play with the
Emotions of strong women
The ticking, in my head
Mentally, a bomb waiting to
Explode
Waves crashing against the rocks
Subtle solitude
My home

---

*When women take on wifely duties but are denied the title of wife by game-playing men!

Excerpted from *To Be: My Spiritual Journey of Finding My Authentic Self*   Signed copies available by sending $20 to Cashapp$darbeauty74 or paypal.me/Dragonflykizz and enter your mailing address as a note with your payment. (PayPal orders may take up to 21 days)

Healing

Many nights
I have cried
I cried rivers
Tonight I cried an ocean
Just from the worship of you
I cried for your unfailing love
Your arms of comfort
In my many nights,
Days, years of darkness
Tonight I cried from
Your healing touch
Thank you LORD, FOR YOUR POWER
Thank you Lord for your angels
That come to my aide
I thank you today for how
You designed me
Truly in love with you
Lavished love that moves me
Your spirit that guides me
That fuels me to keep going
Thank you for grooming, pruning
Molding me

Most of all for all you have embedded in me
I am beautiful
I am healed
I am delivered
Most of all I am in love with
The way you designed
Me!!!
I am amazing because of your
Hands that gave me life!
Honoring you
For my newly love of all of me
I am humbly grateful
But I am so
Happy and excited for my newfound
Capabilities designed by you
I am truly happy and free
Loving all of me
Delighted in this blissful journey
And test of great measure
Greatness!!! All from you
And my determination to
NEVER GIVE UP!!!
Yes Lord, my soul says yes!!!
Designed to be
Loving my destiny!!!!

Excerpted from *To Be: My Spiritual Journey of Finding My Authentic Self*   Signed copies available by sending $20 to Cashapp$darbeauty74 or paypal.me/Dragonflykizz and enter your mailing address as a note with your payment. (PayPal orders may take up to 21 days)

Reflections

Beautiful reflections of my life pass in my
mind,
The hardships,
The pains by divine design,
I am content! Life is falling in line,
No more borrowed time,
I smile,
I breathe,
You live in me,
Bye to the me I used to be,
I see the divine me I was meant to be,
Love for the life divinely created for me,
I am at peace, see?
I love you for loving me,
But mostly because you never left me,
This time I cry for joy I feel,
My labor wasn't in vain,
The clouds fade, the sun shines,
But the fire that burns is blossoming into a
raging glorious light,
Faith in you,
Loving all the beautiful parts of me,
I love the fire and flame brightly shining
from thee.
Hats off to the glorious me!

Excerpted from *To Be: My Spiritual Journey of Finding My Authentic
Self*   Signed copies available by sending $20 to
Cashapp$darbeauty74 or paypal.me/Dragonflykizz and enter your
mailing address as a note with your payment. (PayPal orders may take
up to 21 days)

Quotes from Laile Wilson

experiences on my journey

we are not human beings
we are spiritual experience
we are spiritual beings
having a human experience
I choose to use my spirituality
to make it through this narcissistic
world of chaos destruction
shame and pain.
traumas my friend, no more
emotional intelligence is the way
free to be me

we live in a society of dumping using abusing
with controlling way of manipulation and deceit.
not healing releasing
growing and knowing our authentic self

Copies of *To Be: My Spiritual Journey of Finding My Authentic Self*
available through Amazon at http://mybook.to/ToBe

Author Spotlight

Laile Wilson

Laile Wilson is a 46-year-old single mother of three kings and one princess. She has two grandchildren. She is a proud mother of a college graduate, two gold medalists of basketball at the Giant Stadium, as well as an adoptive mother and caregiver to many. Laile has served as a caregiver and adoptive parent to her three nieces and her nephew. Children in York, Baltimore, New York, and beyond lovingly refer to her as Mom Dukes.

Laile provides emotional support and advocacy for friends and relatives with chemical imbalances (mental health). She served as a Poor People's Foundation volunteer activist for five years and volunteered at Weary Performing Arts Group. She stepped down from her previous profession due to two major heart surgeries.

The first of these surgeries in 2010 started her journey, and after the implantation of a pacemaker and defibrillator in 2018, she started taking classes and going deeper into her natural talent for. Her newest venture is Sacred Water Intuitive Blends. She is also a Master Reiki Healer and teacher.

Laile has performed poetry at The Rooted Collective, the Silken Literary Tent and Ironic.

To Be: My Spiritual Journey of Finding My Authentic Self, is her first book, a collection of poems, available on Amazon. Many more poems and books are in the creating!

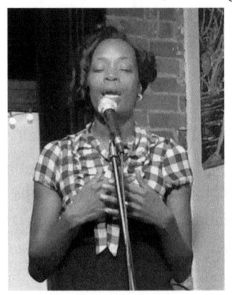

To Be showcases Laile's vulnerability, her transference of negative energy and generational curses, and her survival in a narcissistic world of false narratives, labels, traumas, pains, and anguish. *To Be* serves as testimony of what the mind can do if the foundation is steadfastly set on the positivity of one's owns spiritual development. It showcases how Laile hones her skills to rise above an abusive past. Grab a copy today at http://mybook.to/ToBe and see how it includes and inspires you! Love, peace, be blessed.

Sacred Water Intuitive Blends (herbal tea)
Laiwilsom1536@gmail.com
717-758-7110 (please leave a message)

For signed copies of the book directly from Laile, please send $20 to Cashapp$darbeauty74 or paypal.me/Dragonflykizz and enter your mailing address as a note with your payment. (PayPal orders may take up to 21 days)

My Four Truths of Reflexology
Leslie Punt

I am no stranger to the healing and definitely life-changing power of alternative medicine. My foray into healing mind, body and soul through holistic therapies began with my using hypnosis to treat PTSD symptoms. One of many amazing holistic treatments I tried; it was this that started my quest to learn as much as possible about holistic medicine. I wanted to be able to share this information with those around me who were also in need. So, jump ahead about 20 years... now a certified Full Body Reflexologist and Hypnotist, licensed Aesthetician, Usui Reiki Master Instructor and Holistic Health Coach and CHI sponsor as co-owner of The Center of Balance, LLC., located in Greencastle, Pennsylvania.

Despite having all of this education, knowing many ways to support others; and even more to my surprise... I have found my niche as a Reflexologist. I would never have imagined that I would be working on people's feet one day. One would think that having personally had reflexology would be the reason I was drawn to it, but no... I actually didn't experience reflexology until I became certified in this wonderful healing art. For me, this transformation actually began during the course of my studies; when I discovered that Reflexology kept coming up as a potential solution to so many physical problems within and throughout the body. I was definitely drawn to the thought that this one alternative medicine could make such a difference in our physical self. I definitely needed to learn more about this therapy; so I took my first class in foot reflexology and was forever hooked. My first truth about reflexology was formed: *"One must be grounded to the earth to be able to reach up to the sky."*

Reflexology can be misunderstood; some consider it to be massage of the feet and legs. Others think it is some kind of foot manipulation but not sure how it can work. But to many, it just seems implausible that it can resolve a problem area that is somewhere else in your body, so it must be quackery of sorts! After all, how can one fix a pain in the shoulder or back just by manipulating certain spots located somewhere on your feet? How and why does reflexology work? Similar to acupuncture and acupressure; there are twelve energy meridians located throughout the body – the energy pathways which "Qi" (our energy lifeforce) flows throughout the body. When there is discord located somewhere in the body, it causes imbalance. These imbalances manifest in specific areas on the feet; perhaps as a sore spot, a swelling, a thickness to the tissue and can even manifest physically such as with crystal deposits. My second truth about reflexology was defined: *"A tree is as strong as its roots."*

But Reflexology is not just about working the feet; it also involves working on the body's skeletal systems. Based on the premise that "everything is connected"- when one system is impacted, it affects every other part of the body in some way; i.e. *the foot bone is connected to the ankle bone, is connected to the leg bone, is connected to the thigh bone, is connected to the hip bone and so on!* Body reflexology supports the body as a whole and is a wonderful tool; used to realign each skeletal system, resolve muscular imbalance and detoxify the body. I like to describe it as a cross between acupuncture without the needles, acupressure, healing touch, massage and foot reflexology all mixed together. To my many clients using reflexology to realign and adjust imbalances; it is considered a necessity they just cannot live without. My third truth about reflexology was learned: *"Plant the tree properly and it will grow."*

As a Reflexologist, I use many tools to identify potential problems which help to correct imbalance and deficiencies. Tools like "footprinting" can reflect potential problem areas which can be shown as missing parts of the footprint such as toes, jagged edges and even double print lines to specific areas of the feet. It is important to understand these imbalances in the print and how they can reflect discord that impacts the body. Being able to facilitate necessary changes to correct deficiencies before they become chronic illness is a big key to staying healthy. Detoxification is another tool I use which helps to keep our body systems functioning properly by helping to remove toxins. I rely on Himalayan salt as a natural part of the detox process to safely pull out toxins being released from the body in reflexology by brushing and drumming. Some words used by clients to describe their feelings after foot and body reflexology treatments include "light", "airy", "balanced", "relaxed", "calm" and "whole". Which brings me to my fourth and final truth about reflexology: "*Reflexology; a reflection of true self*".

Reflexology for me; is about sharing the knowledge I have with others to make a difference in their lives. It can be so rewarding to watch the transformation a client goes through as you help them to understand the physical impact both physical and mental stressors have on their body and teach them ways to take better care of themselves. Taking care of the physical helps facilitate healing from within... the mind, body, soul connection is the ultimate pathway to making one whole.

Author Spotlight
Leslie Punt

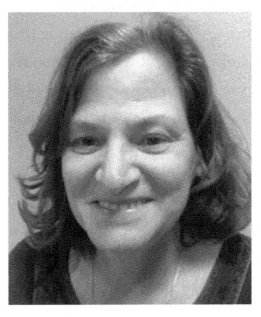

Leslie Punt is co-owner of The Center of Balance, LLC with her twin sister Louise Kemper; and it is located at 29 N Jefferson Street, Greencastle, PA 17225, officially established as a wellness business on March 1, 2018. Her career as a Holistic Practitioner began in 2009 at Holistic Health Associates, Frederick MD; as an Aesthetician, Consulting Hypnotist and a Usui Reiki Master, Leslie is a certified Full Body Reflexologist and graduate of the American College of Healthcare Sciences, with a diploma in Holistic Health Practice with Honors. Her desire is to bring her knowledge and these invaluable services to her clients to help them facilitate optimum health and wellness in all aspects of their lives.

The Center of Balance, LLC current offerings include healing modalities of Foot and Body Reflexology, Reiki,

Hypnosis with Coaching, Massage, Skincare Consulting, arts and classes, and is a very unique artisan gift shop.

The Mirror: From Ashamed to Powerful
Kerri Hample

I grew up hearing,

"She has such a pretty face."

"It's a shame she can't control her weight."

"I wonder if her parents even care."

"Will she ever amount to anything?"

While on a record winning swim relay,

"Wow, she's fast for her size."

In marching band,

"I'm not sure we have a uniform to fit her."

I finished high school weighing 222 pounds and gained another twenty-plus in college.

I truly believed my genetic code pre-destined me to a life where I was not in control of my weight. I started different "programs" around the age of thirteen. I would lose a few and then gain it all back plus some, further convincing myself that "large" was my destiny.

A friend dragged me to yet another "program" when I was twenty-two and for some reason that one stuck. I lost thirteen pounds in the first week and one hundred within one year! I still don't really know why that program worked and others didn't, other than one reason. I had recently moved out on my own and for the first time in my life I was in complete control of what I ate and what I didn't. I could make my own food choices, consistently. While I did lose weight, a lot of it, I developed a very unhealthy relationship with food. If I ate something that was considered "bad" I would run five to ten miles to "get rid of it," or worse, rid myself of it other ways. I was scared to death to return to the overweight version of myself and punished myself for years.

It wasn't until recently (almost twenty years after beginning my weight loss journey) that I experienced the real transformation. Even fifteen years after losing all that weight, I would still look in the mirror and see the "fat girl with the pretty face." As a size eight, I would go to the store and pull size sixteen clothes off the rack and be shocked when they didn't look right. I would wind up at stores that only sell plus-sized clothing. Seems ridiculous, I know!

Why do I share my story? It's certainly not for attention, I've had plenty of that in my life, and it's my least favorite thing! I share because I know I am not alone. Many, many more teens and young women need to know that they have a choice. They also need to know that the transformation is not about pounds lost, it's about mindset shift and happiness gained. I know that many people believe that their health is genetically dictated. You see I proved it wrong ---- you can change your health! You can be smaller, but what's more important is that you are healthier in mind, body and spirit.

I found functional medicine and Arbonne in 2017, a true gift, and I have never looked back. As an educated professor of Occupational Therapy, I went back to school to learn more about functional medicine. Functional medicine, of which I am a certified coach, helps you find the root cause for health issues. Lifestyle changes can make a huge impact on both physical and mental health. I'll spare on the details of my own, let's just say that bread and I are not friends!

I am healthier at forty-three than I was at five, ten, twenty or thirty. I have maintained my hundred-pound weight loss, reversed early stages of ovarian cancer, stabilized my anxiety/depression and my blood sugar, reversed food sensitivities and helped hundreds of people start their journey to being the best version of themselves.

Since finding functional medicine, my goal has always been to include my family and friends on my health journey without forcing them. While functional medicine gave me the tools I needed to get healthy, Arbonne taught me confidence and gave me tools to include others.

If you had asked me even two years ago if I would be comfortable sharing this story or even telling others that I lived this story, I would tell you, you are crazy! Now, thanks to functional medicine and Arbonne my family and I are healthy, strong and living our best lives. That overweight girl that was so ashamed of herself can proudly say:

"Thank you," when someone compliments her because she finally believes them.

"I belong."

"I know how to put food in its place: it's simply energy, information, medicine and connection."

"I amount to more than I ever dreamt possible and I'm just getting started."

The journey to being my best self is ongoing and exciting. Healthy is a state of body and mind and when you do the work on both you can be proud. I am now proud of that young girl because she fought hard to be loved and to love herself. The lessons that I learned growing up taught me and shaped me. I don't wish those experiences on my worst enemy, but I do celebrate her for surviving and now thriving. Those experiences shaped me and led me to a life filled with promise. I'm excited to see how many more people I can support and help discover their power and their health.

Author Spotlight
Kerri Hample

Dr. Kerri Hample is an Occupational Therapist and Certified Functional Medicine Health Coach. She graduated from Thomas Jefferson University in 2000 with a Bachelor of Science in Occupational Therapy and graduated with a clinical doctorate in Occupational Therapy from Rocky Mountain University of Health Professions. In 2009 she completed a certificate in health coaching from the Functional Medicine Health Coaching Academy and completed international certification.

She is currently an Associate Professor of Occupational Therapy at Elizabethtown College and has a private health coaching practice where she is a Regional Vice President with Arbonne International.

In her spare time you can find her and her husband watching two awesome and amazing kids play baseball and compete in all start cheer.

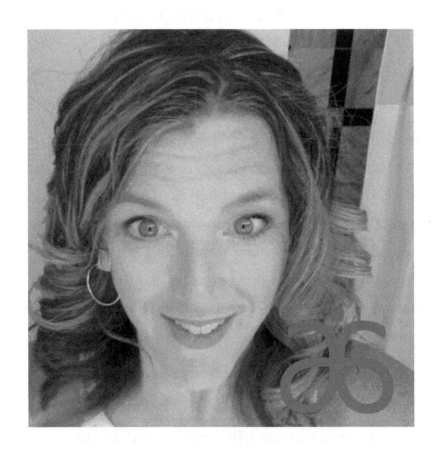

Reach out to her at

717-361-1172

gutfeelingOT@gmail.com

For the Love of Reiki
Katye Anna Clark

My love affair with Reiki began over twenty-five years ago. I was lying on the floor during a workshop when suddenly I felt something I had never felt in this life. The two workshop presenters were doing energy work on me. Suddenly I felt a warm sensation moving through my entire body. One woman had her hand on my heart chakra. The other woman had her hands on my feet. They told me to take deep breaths and as I did, warm energy moved through my entire body. In that moment I felt safe, connected and loved.

That evening I received a healing and my life has never been the same.

I found out later the energy that surged through my body and mind was Reiki. The two women who had given me Reiki told me they would be teaching a Reiki Level One class in a few weeks. I was hooked.

I'll never forget that first Reiki class.

I learned that Reiki is a Japanese healing art that was synthesized into being by Mikao Usui in the late 1800's in Japan. Mikao Usui was a devout Buddhist, who, in his intense desire to understand and work with methods of medicine and healing, developed Reiki. "Reiki" is a Japanese word for the concept: "Universal Life Energy."

Reiki is transferred to the student by a Reiki Master during an attunement process. For many the Reiki attunement is a powerful spiritual experience. My Reiki Master Jackie told us to open up to Reiki. I'll never forget those first attunements. Unlike many in the class I must admit I didn't have a deeply moving spiritual experience. I did however know that Reiki spoke to my heart.

The Reiki Master told us that the most important person we would ever touch was our self. I took what I had learned during that Reiki class and began what has continued as a love affair with Reiki.

I have given myself a Reiki session every day since I was first attuned. As a Reiki Master I have attuned others to Reiki. I have used Reiki on my children and grandchildren. I have used Reiki to help women during childbirth. I've used Reiki after pre, and post opt surgery. I've used Reiki on clients as they were receiving Chemotherapy. I have used Reiki to help people relax as they birth into spirit. As a Master Teacher of Reiki, I was honored to attune my mother to Reiki. At the age of 94 she continues to give herself Reiki every day.

Reiki is more than a healing modality. It's a way of life. Master Usui introduced The Reiki Precepts as a way to bring change into the daily lives of his students. He required his students to meditate on the precept in the morning and at night so that the meaning of the words deepened within them and helped them on their spiritual path.

The Reiki Precepts[15] *by Usui Sensi Roho*

The secret art of inviting happiness
The miraculous medicine of all diseases

Just for today, do not anger.
Do not worry and be filled with gratitude.
Devote yourself to your work.
 Be kind to people.
Every morning and evening,
Join your hands in prayer.
Pray these words to your heart and chant
these words with your mouth.

The Reiki Precepts remind me every day to invite happiness into my life. Every day I walk with gratitude in my heart that Master Usui gave us the gift of Reiki.

---

[15] https://www.Reikiassociation.net/usui-shiki-ryoho.php

As I've said, since the day Reiki and I first met I've had a love affair with it. I personally believe everyone should be attuned to Reiki. Reiki is intelligent. For me, Reiki comes straight from the heart of God. Simply by placing your hands on yourself or someone else the Reiki dance begins – it's a sacred dance. It's a dance of energy. It's a dance of love.

Simply by using Reiki it will teach you, it will guide you. As a Master Teacher of Reiki, I have witnessed that many students simply don't understand the power of Reiki because it's so simple. If you take time to know Reiki, it will guide you and teach you. The only thing a student of Reiki needs to do is use it. Reiki will do the rest.

As a Master Teacher and student of Usui Reiki Ryoho, I will be forever grateful to Master Usui. His quest those many years ago led him onto a pathway of self-discovery and bringing Reiki onto our planet. Now more than ever I believe we need Reiki. Give yourself the gift of Reiki today.

Author Spotlight
Katye Anna

Katye Anna has a BS in Psychology, has been a Reiki Master and Spiritual Teacher for twenty-five years. She was the founder of Pennsylvania School of Spiritual Healing. She taught alongside her husband Allan Clark until he birthed into spirit in 2014. She is the founder of the Birthing Into Spirit Doula Program. She is an author of eight books including *Soul Love Never Ends, Walking with Angels, Birthing Into Spirit, Tell Them - Messages from the World of Spirit, Conscious Construction of the Soul, The Unraveling,* and *The Three Spiritual Keys,* all available on Amazon and at New Visions Books & Gifts in York, PA.

She is a modern-day mystic and Intuitive Reader. She teaches and inspires her students and clients how to live conscious lives of love.

Katye Anna holds an annual transformational retreat at Mago Retreat Center in Sedona AZ.

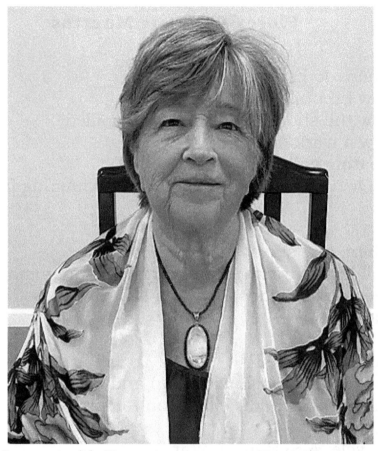

Connect with Katye Anna at www.KatyeAnna.com

Poems of Transition
Annabell Bonilla

Flores Para Los Muertos

Where do I start?
How I rebuilt? How I fell apart?
How the shattered pieces once spilled,
Now a work of art.
Floating with butterflies
   Or running from wolves, and swimming from
                    sharks.

Where do I start?
Childhood drama, like "Word to my momma"
Becomes childhood trauma like no daddy, No
grandma

Pieces borrowed-
The adopted child with pain and sorrow.
The robbed child's effects on tomorrow.

A Cycle, A System, A War
Hamsters on a wheel

Where do I start?
With the Rest In Peaces, that rest in pieces
Sprinkled over wrinkles-- In Time
The best in reasons, the sprinkled seasons
The mingled teasing-- In Mine

Where Do I start?
Rest in peace Jerry and Ricki

And when things got real tricky
Jaiman, Bonk, Shalimar
It still kills Me sickly

Excuse Me if I forget anyone my memory is
Nipsey--
I'm just getting started, so please keep up with Me

Rest In Peace B.R.E. Who became Chozen and
grew
But gone too soon Junie, that burden burned
through
CiCi and Tonya was a double whammy
But Marrcus hit hard and left Me forever clammy

Cano's death made me never want to party
I didn't need to see it
Spare Me the 5 hours-- I'm Sorry
Rigamortis burned in my brain
Bullets, Yelling, Running, Insane
Hug my bestie, It's not a game
PTSD still remains

Julio and Jazzo, straight to the head
Ashanti, My God NO!! Young, Misunderstood,
Misled

A trip to Puerto Rico changed My Life forever
Trick didn't have to go out like that
My friend lost her "Together"

While My kids are older, they too grieve

Rubens death broke My daughter
When they told her he had to leave

So where do I start?
If it will never end
It still continues, A part of US
We're still losing friends.

Ani B.

Some Thing

What I would do for something Real
Not something fake
Not something borrowed
Something true

Something that won't go stale with time
Something that's not shared, it's mine
Something that words cannot describe
Something that flutters like butterflies -inside

Never a feeling of emptiness
Loneliness, regretfulness - sunshine

Warmth, comfort, safe
Longing, waiting, faith
Honest, respectful, true
Funny, sincere, you... Me...

Silence now...
Broken pieces scraping - heartburn

Long nights crying, denying
Trying to forgive and forget
Trying not to regret... time

Lies manipulation, carelessness
Consumed in dirt
Never works
Trust over? ... Maybe

But wanting still...

Unconditional, undestructable
Never blinded, Open minded
Freedom of speech but careful
Considerate, outreach, careful, - Gentle

Reborn again and again - Never dying
Fairytale happy
Why not? I deserve it!

What I would do for something real
Not something fake
Not something borrowed
Something True
Something Mine.

Ani B.

Hope

I don't know, I don't know,
I don't know what it is.
Everybody's taunting Me -But-
They don't know, Cuz I don't know
the reason for Me.
Day in and day out, I think.
Will I make it 2 the end?
We'll see...

I want 2 leave, I want 2 stay
What am I supposed to do?
They keep taking pieces from Me -Cuz-
I'm not whole
I don't know
Just how my heart beats.
I try to fight back, It stings
I'm stronger and wiser now
So things...

Will come together, Brand new weather
Yes the sun will shine
Morning clouds drift away slowly -I-
Think I'm fine
Finally happy to be Me.
I have grown, my heart sings.
Accepted I'll grow old
And die someday...

Ani B.

A.N.I.

Cancer Baby Moon Child
Loving, Loyal, Nurturing, Emotional
Lanc Lanc, Stank Stank
5 Bros, 0 Sisters, 2nd to Youngest
SELF- Raised
Illegitimate Foster Child
Black, White, Spanish, Cambodian
Content Outsider
Successful Flunky
Street and Book Smart
Teen Mom- Growing Mom
Ex-Cartel
Punching Bag, Foot Stool, Stepping Stone
Sunshine, Energy, Purpose, Force
Wrung out Mr Clean Healer
Da Glue
Healthy Living Foods LLC
TransitionS
All they Titis
Holistic Health Coach
Shattered Master-Peace

TransitionS For Every Body

People put so much emphasis on the ending
result.
They discourage themselves before they begin.

TRANSITION is hope.
And with one step,
the goal begins to feel more and more attainable.
Where the struggle was,
is eventually replaced with education and routine.
Hunger for knowledge grows due to results.

TRANSITION is embraced.
You knew it would be tough,
But you took on the challenge.
You took the first step
Then the second.
Always remembering it
And respecting it
Because You too
Were once in a different stage of Transition.

-Ani B.

My Transition
Annabell Bonilla

Annabell Bonilla, born June 26, 1985, was raised in Lancaster City, Pennsylvania. The second to youngest and only girl with five brothers, fitting in wasn't the easiest. She spent early years in the streets or writing and caring for her pets. Despite a rough childhood with constant uprooting, and becoming a teen mom in 2003, Annabell graduated from Buehrle's Alternative School, in Lancaster, in 2004. Upon graduating, Annabell was invited to present her writings to fellow students. Poetry was the inspiration behind her growth, and she became a youth advocate and a mentor in a school known for misfits.

Annabell routinely fell into leadership roles in the workforce, too. Working in factories to support her daughter, she always felt misplaced. She wanted to do more. Annabell eventually made her way to York in the summer of 2006, where she met Erick Negron, with whom she formed a partnership.

Her daughter's father Marrcus had been dealing with severe complications from his diabetes for a few years. He passed away November 14, 2008, on World Diabetes Day.

Annabell's son Erick Jr. was born in March 2009. Determined to keep pushing for her family, Annabell enrolled and graduated from YTI Career institute in 2010 with an Associates in Dental Assisting. Most of her career in dental assisting was devoted to pediatric dentistry.

Annabell obtained her certification to present Oral Health Education and continued to expand her knowledge. After years of learning the dental office, Annabell took a break and loaded trucks. In a slump, she bounced around ideas, wanting something that would incorporate her experience and hunger for teaching and presentation. She needed to be available for her children but the need to work consumed her. She went back to dental assisting due to the flexible schedule, but her hunger remained. An empty feeling remained. No amount of money, no empty bottle, no group of people could fill it. She lived to raise her children but became less present due to working. More issues brewed. More insecurities with herself with barriers from past trauma deflected progress.

Helping Erick with his Healthy Living Foods events and presentations in her free time, Annabell found light in helping others. She found happiness in the creativity of decorating and the appreciation to her energy was inspiring. But after a freak accident in October 2018, Annabell was not able to return to work normally. Her entire perspective on her purpose had been altered.

Derailed, shifted, and shattered, she fought to put it all back together. Her mindset had always been of one that was damaged by her own traumas and she consumed herself in making her second chance count. Healing not just on the outside but within.

Changing eating habits, toxic lifestyle practices, and educating herself on some of her own hurdles and roadblocks, she transitioned from the hurt caterpillar to the Beautiful Monarch Butterfly. All the while, still jumping hurdles, but allowing the transparency in her flaws to show her genuineness. Motivating without judgement, she continued to grow forward, committing to understand with an open mind.

Healthy Living Foods, now in York and surrounding cities, has opened the door to an outside box of uncharted opportunities. Determined to expand and grow the purpose, Annabell is now the Event Coordinator for Healthy Living Foods LLC and Owner of TransitionS For Every Body LLC, a produce store with the hopes of cheffing up Vegetarian Latin Food and potentially advancing to a Mobile Food Truck in order to reach people through food, desserts, and beyond.

Intertwining her knowledge in oral care, self-care, and nutrition, Annabell began expanding her HLF branches with projects like her "World Diabetes Day for M. Kiss" – a Holistic Event dedicated to her daughter's dad, Marrcus

Pack, and "JDRF Walk For A Cure- Team HLF For M. Kiss". "United Diasporas" is also a project in process for 2020. Annabell offers classes and presentations on basic skills and steps in transitioning, sometimes using the same poetry from her childhood to resonate with troubled youth and their parents.

Constantly expanding her knowledge, Annabell found great interest in Tarot Reading and the effects of Childhood Trauma. Continuing classes and applying the knowledge to her own self-care, she vowed to help adults and children navigate through some of the same issues she had from a different perspective. Using karaoke and spoken words to break social anxieties, Annabell has run with every dream and opportunity to shine presented, accomplishing more in one year than in the 33 prior. She even created "Anita Bonita" – a character who loves showing her fruit hat and drinking coconuts. This new complete out of the box approach is working.

Annabell now has a stand at the market where she provides fresh, healthy, local and tropical produce and fruit juices. She brings awareness and education to feeding the body, mind and soul. Future plans include children's health books, a collaborated poetry book with her daughter and Urban Farm Interviews. She has interest in presenting her poetry globally and is studying to be a Holistic Health Coach and Nutritionist. She loves spending time with her daughter Samarrah, her son Erick Jr, and her two-year-old Jack Russell Terrier Bornelle. She also loves cooking, singing and listening to music, and Spanish dancing. She hopes to share her energy and light to those in dark places. Using her trauma as experience, she continues to pay it forward.

Author Spotlight
Annabell Bonilla

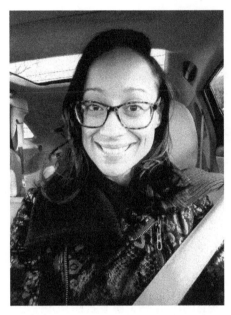

Owner of Transitions For Everybody LLC- Supporting Your Transition - Body, Mind, & Soul

annabell.bonilla@yahoo.com

I: anita.bonita717

FB: HLF - TransitionS

717-332-9986

The Key to Transformation
John Stewart

When you picture a hypnotist, maybe you imagine some vaguely evil villain swinging a pocket watch in front of a victim's eyes. But hypnotism is actually a wonderful tool used by trained therapists to try to reach and relax your mind in a different kind of way.

My first encounter with hypnosis occurred many years ago. When I was a teen and young adult I struggled severely with stuttering. At this age, perhaps you can imagine the social ramifications this would cause a person. Despite the efforts of a well-meaning speech pathologist, I continued to stutter. In a fit of desperation, I sought the help of a local hypnotherapist. A hypnotherapist is a therapist who uses hypnosis to help his/her clients.

My meetings with him were the most relaxing 60 minutes I've ever enjoyed. The stuttering didn't disappear overnight but the bottom line that I quickly learned from those first hypnosis sessions were that this stuttering was something that I was doing and had control over. I was choosing to stutter and since I had control over the stuttering I could make a change of mindset. Looking back now, it seemed so simple a process but getting that message across to the subconscious mind was the key. The hypnotist convinced my deeper subconscious mind to relax when speaking. Over a period of weeks, I began to speak controllably, more relaxed and eventually with fluidity.

The idea of hypnosis as someone controlling minds is outdated. Really, the opposite is true. Yes, it's a vulnerable feeling to let someone else guide you through a less guarded realm of your consciousness. But in reality, the hypnotherapist will only go into subjects that you want to delve into.

The hypnotherapist has the professional skills to allow your mind to relax and reveal some of the deeper roots or meanings to our problems. Plus, the hypnotherapist will perform some demonstrations to give you an idea of how the subconscious mind works, as well as how you can expect the rest of the session to go. No matter what happens, you are in the lead the whole time.

The state of deep relaxation, in which you find yourself, during a hypnotherapy session, can vary depending on a number of factors. But one thing is always true: you won't be asleep. Yes, your mind will be in a state of great relaxation, but that's not the same as drifting off under the covers at night. The hypnotherapist is merely suggesting a change in feeling, behavior, and perception of yourself and your surroundings.

You have already experienced the state of hypnosis many times in your life. If you've ever gone to a movie theater and got wrapped up in the plot of the film's story you were in effect hypnotizing yourself. You are believing that the images on the screen are real despite the fact that you knew, consciously, the actors are well paid professionals and the backdrops are often in a movie studio backlot in Hollywood.

Bypassing the critical thinking of our conscious minds and suggesting new ideas to the subconscious mind is in essence what hypnosis is all about. Since hypnosis can reach the subconscious directly without our logical thoughts or defenses getting in the way, it can break those negative cycles. So, sometimes it's necessary to go into a trance to get out of a trance. Sure, that sounds pretty weird, but the basic idea of bypassing your logical mind to get the roots of your unwanted behavior is compelling.

Many notable people have used hypnosis to make changes and improvements in their life. Matt Damon quit smoking as a direct result of hypnosis and has been quoted as saying, "It's the best decision I've ever made." James Earl Jones and Bruce Willis quit stuttering. Tiger Woods improved his concentration on the golf course.

So, if you're thinking of trying out hypnotherapy, but aren't sure what to expect, here's what really happens when you see a hypnotherapist. You are in control.

If you choose to see a hypnotherapist, your appointment will begin a lot like a regular therapy session. You'll go into an office, then sit down and talk with the therapist about what you'd like to achieve in the session. Whether you're looking to reduce pain, deal with stress and anxiety or modify or eliminate a behavior you will communicate that to your hypnotherapist so they can figure out the best way to help you. You, the client, are the one who is in control. As a hypnotherapist, my role is to serve as your tour guide. You decide where we go. My job is just to get you there.

Author Spotlight

John Stewart

John Stewart is the Susquehanna Valley's Health Hypnotherapist and a member of the National Guild of Hypnotists, NGH. He is certified in the specialized procedure of Virtual Gastric Band weight management hypnosis. John has been a Clinical Hypnotherapist since 2011 and established Lancaster Hypnotherapy in 2015. The office of Lancaster Hypnotherapy offers a comfortable, professional and relaxing atmosphere. It is located conveniently in downtown Lancaster city, with off street parking and ADA access.

John is a life-long resident of Lancaster County and is a perpetual student. His interests in human consciousness and potentials delves beyond hypnosis. Spoon bending workshops, for example, allow participants to experience their own unique abilities. John has a penchant for travel, having visited three continents. When not traveling, he can be found under the starry skies at night with his large telescope named Dream Weaver.

LancasterHypnotherapy.com-

717-340-3100.

313 West Liberty Street, Suite 129,

Lancaster, PA 17603

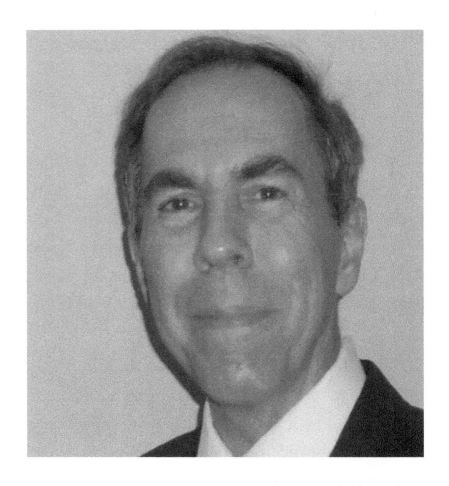

John Stewart

LancasterHypnotherapy.com-

717-340-3100

My Journey from Health Helper to Holistic Health Coach
Rebecca Johnston

I am honored to share part of my journey that led me to becoming a holistic health and functional medicine health coach with you! I have always loved the word "journey." A simple definition of this word is "an act of traveling from one place to another." We often think of travel as using some mode of transportation to get from point A to point B.

For example, when we plan a trip or a long-awaited family vacation, we may need to put in time planning to make sure things are "just right." Some may find this stressful but hopefully in the end, it is all worth it. We can then look back and pat ourselves on the back for doing the work to make sure things turned out right and that we have fantastic memories of that time.

I believe there is much more to our personal journeys than simply getting from point A to point B. A personal journey is much more meaningful. If we look at a personal journey over someone's lifetime, I believe it is something that happens naturally as we grow, develop and have more life experience. Sometimes it takes a little retrospection.

Although some of us may be adept at recognizing what we want to accomplish early on in life and progressing toward that end, others may take life more naturally and learn how we really feel about it and our place in it as we go.

I believe that each way of being in the world is equally fine. For me to write out my "journey of transformation" with a holistic modality, it helps to be clear about how I think about the meaning of a journey.

When looking back from where I am now (point B but still traveling), I can see why I am here. This was not always the case. I spent many years feeling a bit "lost" regarding the direction of my journey. I cannot genuinely share my story without revisiting my childhood where my father had the chronic disease diabetes mellitus and experienced many complications, including two kidney transplants and much more. He was insulin-dependent, and as a CPA and attorney by profession, he was quite meticulous in tracking his health and blood sugar numbers. He was adept at knowing which type of food he needed at which specific time or which food he needed to stay away from to prevent a diabetic reaction. Insulin fluctuations can cause rapid changes in mood and behavior and he always did his best to maintain the status quo.

To this end, I was his "health helper" from the very start. I was always on alert to what the next need was. If I needed to run to grab a banana, crackers or insulin bottle,

I was ready. It was our "norm." I am not complaining or feeling sorry for myself. I believe all things happen for a reason.

My father lived a good life with many accomplishments. He passed away suddenly in his sleep at age 61 on a sleep apnea machine, after a bout of needing to take more insulin in the middle of the night. Needing more insulin was fairly "normal" so it is still a bit of a mystery. However, losing my Dad so suddenly at the time, right after my college graduation, was a big contributor on my personal journey.

I had majored in psychology in college, absolutely loved what I had learned and always wanted to apply this in a profession. I ended up working in healthcare in various medical offices as I moved around for my husband's position. It was not until after having my beloved son and experiencing my own health issues that I did seem to "wake up" and set my sights anew on my path.

Something very distant but familiar woke up in me. As much as I tried to push it away at times, it would not leave me. It was reminding me of what I have always known. I **love** and **need** to help people! I have been a "health helper" from childhood and chose psychology because I was intrinsically drawn to it. I was reminded of all the times I felt helpless as a girl, watching my Dad suffer and how different foods affected him. There is more to food than simply tasting good and filling our stomachs. The seeds were planted in me as I grew up.

I did not understand, as I do now, that food is information. Food breaks down and serves a higher purpose. Everything we consume becomes us, through our cells and bloodstream. God made us this way for a reason. Everything in nature is connected. If we take the time to nourish ourselves mindfully and understand what we are consuming, instead of treating food as a "quick fix to hunger", we can become healthier, stronger and heal our own bodies and minds. We can potentially live longer with a higher quality of life as we age in years.

After my own health started to crash, which involved symptoms from different body systems and MANY visits to "specialists", all of which could not really help me, I woke up even more. This "rude awakening" and inconvenience in my life, combined with the memories of my dad's experience, along with what I already knew and loved about psychology, is what got me to my current point B on my journey.

I enrolled in the Institute of Integrative Nutrition, immersed myself into learning again, and became certified as an Integrative Nutrition Health Coach. It felt amazing! They teach a concept that I will always revere called "Primary Foods", which includes other aspects of health such as Spirituality, Relationships, Career and Finances.

Food that we consume is considered "Secondary Food." After all, although I am an advocate for eating whole, clean foods now, I know we can eat all the broccoli we want, but it will not improve our overall wellness. If we get up every day dreading going to work, have no close friends to trust and support us, have nothing in our bank account for security and feel no true drive and purpose in life, we will be unwell.

I realized my own need for more support and accountability with my health goals. I obtained the services of my own personal health coach for a time. I learned more about food labels, grocery stores and eating organic. I started eating whole foods and cut out processed foods. No more diet drinks or artificial sweeteners that just upset gut health. I cut way back on sugar, dairy and gluten to lower inflammation.

I incorporated "superfoods" and learned about macronutrients. I added more movement, exercise and Mother Nature into my day. I started using doTERRA pure essential oils and used non-toxic products to cut down on man-made chemicals that lead to health issues of all sorts.

I completed a course on environmental toxins (talk about an eye opener!) and earned a Women's Health Certification where I learned even more about the immune system, hormonal systems and functional nutrition as it relates to female health. I was beginning to feel something I never felt before and that feeling was "empowered."

Feeling empowered with my new healthier lifestyle and certifications, I set my sights on how I can spread this joy and wellness lifestyle to others. I searched my soul for a meaningful name for my holistic health coaching practice. I was drawn back to one of my favorite concepts in psychology, which is the lifelong debate over Nature versus Nurture. That is, what is the extent to which aspects of our behavior are influenced by genetic factors (Nature) or acquired through outside influences such as our environment (Nurture)? Since I was combining psychology and nutritional wellness and wishing to help others find what really nourishes them in **all** ways including my love for Nature, I would call my practice "Nature & Nourish Wellness." So that felt complete.

I began seeing personal clients and facilitated seasonal whole foods detoxes that cut out inflammatory foods for just five days so it felt achievable and I received positive feedback. After my first session with my first client, I remember feeling so happy and fulfilled in a way that I never felt. It was clear that health coaching would not be "just another job" to me, but something I felt passionate about and would actually do for free, albeit we all have to make a living. Why not do something I love to do that actually serves people?

Since I love to learn and dig deeper, I have now earned the title Functional Medicine Certified Health Coach after completing a year-long certification from The Functional Medicine Coaching Academy, the only school directly affiliated with The Institute of Functional Medicine. This curriculum dives deep into positive psychology, mind-body medicine and the potential to partner with IFM-trained practitioners who look for the root cause of disease through a holistic perspective and systems biology.

I am trained in techniques such as Motivational Interviewing which serves to help people discover their own deeper motivations and vision where I gently guide them in a client-centered fashion. This field is growing exponentially as it is seeing amazing results with patients finding answers they could not find elsewhere. If I can play even a small role in the support of those suffering through real health challenges, I will have lived a purposeful life.

I hope this, in some way, is an inspiration to you on your own journey, whatever path you are on! There may be times when you feel bewildered, sad, helpless or insecure along the way. Hang in there because we never know where that path will naturally take us. I have learned that we do NOT have to remain feeling unhealthy, helpless, uninspired and unmotivated. We are made to grow and transform. We are stewards of the very bodies and minds that are entrusted to us. We have the power within to decide what to eat, what toxins we eliminate, how much sleep we get, who we spend time with, what our spiritual life is like, what career path to take or redirect and how much quality time we spend in nature. We are in control of our own nourishment from this beautiful land called Earth.

If you hear a nagging internal voice, consider quieting your mind and listening to it. Where could it lead you on your journey? Let it in. Let it empower you. Take the necessary steps to reach your point B. If you feel you cannot quite achieve your goals on your own, then perhaps seeking out a qualified health and wellness coach or other professional would be a step in the right direction. No one need feel alone on their journey. And remember to always keep moving forward.

Author Spotlight
Rebecca Johnston

I provide services that inspire mind, body and spirit nourishment. I work **with** my clients to co-create the steps on their journey by offering support, guidance and accountability. I use positive psychology, motivational interviewing, unconditional positive regard, SMART goals and many other holistic "'tools" to help guide my clients to the outcomes they are seeking.

We can work together in various areas of health, including but not limited to, nutrition, movement/exercise, sleep, stress management, emotional wellness, gut health, hormonal health, relationships and spirituality and overall achieving positive habit change.

Specific services include one FREE Discovery Session, individual health coaching sessions (in-person, telephonically or virtually), whole foods detox program, healthy grocery store tour, pantry cleanouts and wellness workshops. I also provide natural solutions to health concerns through education and use on doTERRA essential oils and non-toxic products. FREE doTERRA wellness consult and iTOVi scan available. Will travel regionally.

Rebecca Johnston
Integrative and Functional Medicine Health Coach
Nature & Nourish Wellness
doTerra Wellness Advocate

Websites:

www.naturenourishwellness.com

www.mydoterra.com/rebeccajohnston3

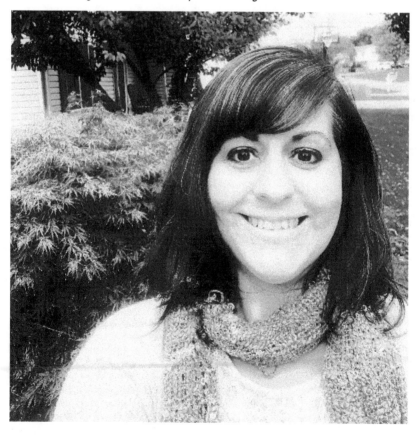

Gratitude Page

The Profound Healing Magic of a Feather and a Flower
Brandy Yavicoli

My personal journey through energy work and shamanism has gone from complex structured deep traditionalism to the simple peaceful magic of a flower.

As my left hand held the Star Jaguar formed of sacred clay, my right hand lifted the pelt-covered stem of the chanupa to my left shoulder. I closed my eyes, no longer seeing the circle of Masters around me, but feeling their collective energy along with the ancestors above us, and the power of the Jaguar Clan through this sacred pipe. I said a prayer of gratitude for the past and of appreciation for everything that brought me to this moment.

I lifted the chanupa to my right shoulder. Signifying the future, I sent a blessing of hope for things to come for us all. We asked that the spirits would hear our song, singing it out loud and sending it into the universe for the love of all, in high vibration, adding our soul signatures to creation.

The tip of the pipe made its way to my forehead. Activating my third eye, I could feel the light of the Star Jaguar penetrating my being and amplifying my own light. "May I sing the Song of the Seekers and embody my mission here on earth."

Opening my eyes, my gaze fell on the Mayan Shaman Elder leading the ceremony. My teacher for the past two months, he sat like a cross-legged laughing Buddha made of heavy mud. Only he wasn't laughing right now. The tone of this Naming Ceremony was one of initiation, and this was serious ancient business.

Touching the end of the long Star Jaguar pipe to my heart center, I said a prayer of the heart. To follow my heart and live from it, with courage and strength. I thanked the ancestors. Putting the wood to my lips, I drew in enough for the sacred smoke to fill my mouth. Letting it out slowly, I could taste the tobacco, sage, mugwort, and other countless herbs that had been added into this blend over the lifetime of this specific Pipe Bearer. I lifted the pipe up to the heavens in reverence, feeling the energy of it in my hands, then down in front of me bowing and touching my forehead to the pelt on the shaft. One more blessing of gratitude and I passed the Star Jaguar to the man on my left.

When I received the talking feather tied with a red string around its base, I closed my eyes once more. Somehow, words didn't seem right. Lifting the large feather

- heavier than it seemed - out in front of me, I took a deep breath and was called to let it out, through the feather, in a powerful long tone filling the room with its resonance. Bowing, I passed the feather to my left. For I had just been named "Ka'lay Molay – Song of the Seeker."

What is the most powerful teaching I gained from those months? The unmistakable power of a feather.

A year later, I lay on Mexican blankets, under the slow melodic beat of a buffalo drum, beside an eight by ten-foot ground altar made of stone, flowers, and sacred objects. The smell of palo santo filled the room and the voice of Mother Earth spoke in between the drums and smoke. It was the voice of my teacher, this time a woman from the Forest of the Columbia Mountains and the Hoh River Valley. A lifetime of studying with Shamans from Siberia, South America, Canada, and Guatemala melted into the voice of the trees and the earth with which she spoke so closely. Her own raw experiences with Nature bled through her aura field and she spoke in a compassionate, ancient cadence of one who knows the rhythms of the Earth and the wisdom of the Rivers. In between her spoken words was the deep call to journey within to our own ancient wisdom, and to hear – and trust - the guidance of our intuition.

She asked us to accept a gift of a flower from the altar, whichever one was calling to us. We placed the flower at heart center and feeling it blessing our Hearts with the miracle of the Great Mystery, with the unconditional, and total love of the Mother, we connected with its beauty, connected to the love of the Earth. Then, we were gently instructed to place the flower to our forehead. There is nothing in this world like a third eye blossoming from a flower — I have no words to do it justice. Returning from the point at which time had flowed into the infinite unfolding of love, we continued the Flower Blessing at different points on the body in gratitude, magic, love, openness, and sacredness.

Over the three years I worked with her, what was the most profound teaching of all? The simple magic of a flower. Shamanic energy work isn't about making a big spectacle, or even having a mind-blowing experience. It is about connecting with and feeling the healing energies of nature; the flowers, feathers, stones, and the channeled energy from the practitioner that awakens more of that within yourself.

When we enter into sacred space, through ceremony or simply by acknowledging the sacredness within and without, we experience the sacred medicine all around us.

I now use feathers and flower blessings in every healing session as we open to the healing magic within and without. I encourage you next time you are in Nature to follow your intuition and receive the blessings of the Earth and Sky, in sacredness, in all the forms they speak to your Soul.

Author Spotlight
Brandy Yavicoli

Brandy Yavicoli, Energy Channel and Shamanic Reiki Master Teacher works alongside your guides to bring you into greater harmony using sound, crystals, nature items such as feathers and flowers, shamanic techniques, divination, energy healing, and personal channeled attunements. Each synergistic session is unique and power-filled with your highest vibrational signature! She offers one-on-one sessions and group trainings out of her home amongst the mountains and orchards of Gardners, PA, from Etheric Connections Crystal Shop and Healing Center in Gettysburg, PA, and through distance work. Check out her website for more information and to connect at

FeedYourSpiritLLC.com
717-451-5505
Brandy@FeedYourSpiritLLC.com
FeedYourSpiritLLC.com

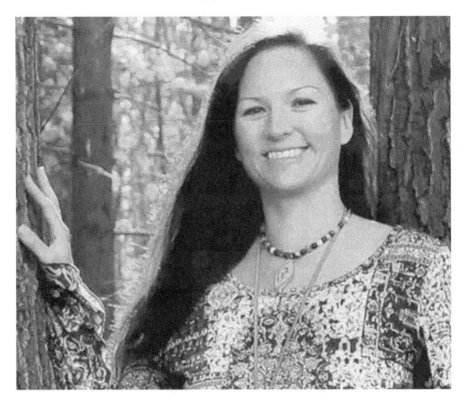

Brandy Yavicoli   Feed Your Spirit LLC

Second Chance Collar
Clint Chronister

Being born into a world into a family that yells, fights, screams and is just out right negative to one another must be hell to a newborn. But that is how my life started. As far back as I can remember, my childhood was hard. Being raised in negativity, I became it. Day in and day out-- parents arguing back and forth, fights, slamming of doors and scuffles. Then it continued in school with the other kids because I was different, being bullied, outcast, and rejected. All twelve years of school were utter hell. Then to add to that, somewhere between the ages of seven and twelve, I was molested by my cousin and my father.

Things I held dear to me were taken from me either through death or destruction. It was hard growing up not knowing my place in the world. Then, church was forced onto me at childhood Sunday school or bible school. I learned quickly about hypocrites then. I started to place resentment towards God for he is the one that gave me life and brought me here to suffer.

Coming into adulthood, life went into the next level. I became a father and that was awesome, feeling that I created something. Imagine later to find out that seven members of my family could have been the possible father as well, like for instance, my stepdad, my father, two of my cousins, and my father's brother-in-law. The betrayal that washed over me was real. Not to mention that before I even found that out, my daughter was taken from me for three years. I didn't know if she was alive or dead until I got a child support summons.

Now, having my kid just disappear on me. Not knowing if she was kidnapped or what was up did something to me mentally and emotionally. I snapped. So, then, I made myself the outcast, a loner. I stayed away from people, hated people. I used them for what I could get out of them to benefit me. I went to work, came home, and just isolated myself from others. I just started studying and researching all kinds of stuff from the occult, mythology, demonology, angelicism, paganism, Christianity, cabalism, paranormal, and the list goes on. I was a walking resentment towards God because I blamed him for all this that went on in my life since birth.

As the years passed, I started to get really sick. I mean downhill fast sick. I went from 250 to 400 pounds sick in six months. The doctors said I had congestive heart failure, that is what caused everything else to go to hell real quick. I gained water weight, got a sort of narcolepsy, could walk but only two or three feet before getting winded and fatigued, it wasn't good.

The doctor performed a heart ablation. It should have been simple in and out, but I woke up three weeks later from a medically induced coma. Now I got God-smacked and karma at the same time.

Going through all that wasn't enough, though. In the beginning, I saw some scary beyond-the-veil stuff. I also witnessed some very awesome and beautiful things as well. Where I went next, I do not ever want to return.

Waking up from the coma was hell, scary — all the above. I was strapped, mitted, and tubed in a bed in the ICU. I couldn't speak. I was restrained. I didn't even know where and what was going on.

The nurse was surprised I was awake. I looked at her, lost and scared, trying to figure out what was going on. She gave me an equally confused face. Then I passed out again. When I woke up again, my mom and daughter and doctors were there, and they told me what happened.

The original surgery had gone well for my heart and they had expected me to go into recovery, but when I came off the anesthesia and the oxygen everything went wrong. My lungs had collapsed, and I had fallen into a coma. It took seven of them to restrain me to get the tube back down my throat and to hook me up to life support. My organs were failing, I had pneumonia three times, I died once for fifteen minutes and the other twenty. I got MRSA somehow.

Now I believe the last time I died, the twenty- minute death, is where I had the choice to ask for forgiveness and go to the light or go to the dark. The beings that were there were wheeling me down to hell I suppose. The beings had doctor coats and they were no headed, bloody limbed, walking on their stub things. They couldn't touch me though. There were millions of them through the darkness coming fast and light above me, so I looked up and woke up from my coma. That, I believe, was my second chance.

Waking from my coma, going from critical to stable condition, and finally getting put in a regular room on recovery was a slow process. It was during this process that change began. Karma happened and I experienced my own darkness in a new way. I believe everything I did to people when I was dark and negative, and all the hate that was going on within me finally caught up and was delivered back to me. I felt the pain and hurt of it all and went through some of it again as well. I felt all that I had inflicted on to others. It didn't feel good at all.

I was completely helpless, but I had to go through those helpless feelings to understand and feel what I was. I cried like a waterfall. I asked God for His forgiveness and I was sorry I blamed Him. Then things started to happen. Recovery got faster. I was finally able to leave the hospital.

My recovery didn't stop because I left the hospital. New life was given to me. I am disabled now. I have to be on two machines and I had to learn how to take care of my tracheostomy. I learned to walk all over again. It was challenging and still is, but I can't have that stop me. I have to find solutions to carry on.

So, I got into the holistic lifestyle and gym, Tai Chi, Zumba. It started to become a routine for me. I started going back to New Visions Bookstore where I have been going now for twenty years.

At New Visions, I've met new people, found a person to teach me Reiki, and even became a Reiki practitioner. I went to a lot of Reiki shares which have helped me heal. I got my Reiki 1 Certification. I also wanted to investigate massage therapy, so I went to school for that. In that clinic, I felt light and love and peace.

The feeling I had come over me was like no other I have ever felt before. I didn't want to leave. It was like all the fears and hates and problems never existed. I was in total bliss and peace and love. It almost felt like I wasn't in my own body or on the planet. It was something special to feel, witness, and be in.

When I felt the bliss, I began my journey into staying in that presence. So, then I figured I would start my own business. The massage thing I still love with a passion, but I don't have all that money for a license and all that tape you must cross. I am just proud of myself that I am certified and know what I am doing.

Then my other calling came out. I am an intuitive artist, portrait reader, and energy healer. My artwork in some shape or form can and will help someone in some fashion. I also handcraft things, from dreamcatchers to smudge feathers and jewelry pendants.

So many wonderful doors and opportunities are still opening for me. Second chances do happen. Mine just came to me as a collar, a reminder I live with, to keep using myself and my art to inspire others and motivate them to not give up. Because I will not give up, I have seen my life go from utter hell to something I would never believe. Yes, it will still be hard, but it is so much better and more rewarding. One of my favorite things to say from experience:

Things that come easy and with hardly any effort are not worth it and are dark and hate — for that is easy. But something you must work for, and strive for, even fight for, is so much more rewarding — that is love and light.

My friends, it is easy to hate. It is harder to show and give love and stay in that light. ***I would rather fight than submit***.

Love and light.

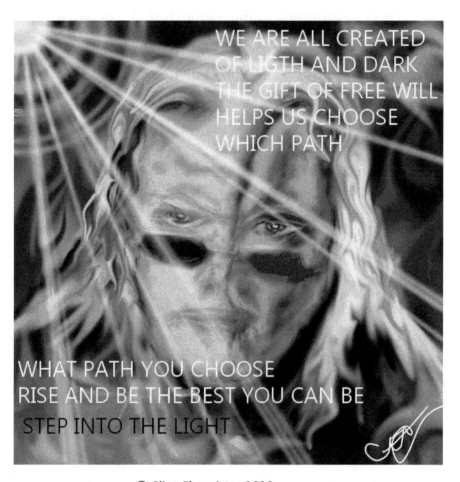

© Clint Chronister 2020

Author Spotlight

Clinton R. Chronister

Clinton R. Chronister is the owner and operator of Phoenixdragonwolf Holistic Healing Arts.

One of his best accomplishments is creating this business. Clint doesn't give up easily and he followed through on making this possible. He is also a Certified Reiki Practitioner and Certified Massage Therapist.

Clint is a very kindhearted, strong willed, empathic, blunt, giving person and a person you can rely on. He does not believe in giving up.

phoenixdragonwolfhha.com

phoenixdragonwolfhha@gmail.com

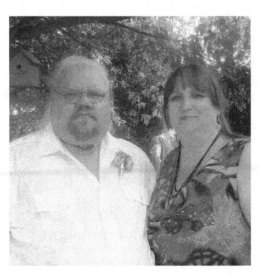

How I Fully Recovered from Complex PTSD
Mary Kalbach

I hope to describe my own experience and introduce you to the tools I used to fully recover from this life-crippling condition because if this describes you, my heart goes out to you. You don't have to live this way! I'm walking, joyfully skipping, grounded, regulated, proof of that!

I honestly don't remember a time in my childhood when I wasn't experiencing some signs and symptoms of a traumatized brain. As a child, young adult, and then young mom I experienced:

- Medical trauma
- Many experiences of sexual abuse of self
- Repeatedly witnessing sexual abuse of someone close to me
- Repeated and prolonged spiritual abuse
- Psychological/emotional abuse
- Emotional neglect
- Continual Retraumatization through parenting adopted kids with trauma history

It wasn't until I was in my thirties and already a mom to many that I was officially diagnosed with Complex PTSD from all of these experiences. I was seeing a wonderfully kind, caring and skillful cognitive ("talk") therapist who was helping me strategize ways to manage the behaviors of our adopted children.

As I worked with that therapist, he helped me to identify the many symptoms I was experiencing as clear markers of well-developed C-PTSD. These symptoms included:

- Vivid, horrifying nightmares that often ended in screaming, thrashing and sometimes inadvertently attempting to harm my husband
- Nearly constant flashbacks - sudden and detailed re-living in my mind past experiences of abuse throughout the day with no warning
- Hyperarousal - constant vigilance and attention to surroundings and sensory information
- Dissociation - near constant state of dissociation, or living outside of my own mind/body
- Pervasive feeling of dread and doom - no felt sense of safety
- Depression and suicidal ideations
- Constant feeling of shame and guilt that lived in my "gut"
- Unpredictable fits of rage that felt highly justified
- Several Physical health issues with no physiological basis (Conversion Disorder)
- Erratic swings from strong, passionate emotions to flat affect and inability to show/receive affection

In other words, I had about every symptom in the book that indicated both PTSD and Complex PTSD.

When those fits of rage became regularly directed toward my husband and children, I was convicted that something had to change. My family had become the unwitting victims of my own childhood abuse. That cycle had to stop. It was simply unacceptable to continue on without caring for my own inner condition and highly destructive outward behaviors.

This journey was not easy. It took many years, some financial commitment, a huge dose of humility, and lots and lots of self-reflection and willingness to doggedly dive into the most difficult experiences of my life. I was dedicated to getting better and willing to try just about anything to make that happen. My family was worth it. I was worth it!

As much as I loved and respected that cognitive therapist, after ten years I hadn't made a whole lot of progress in actually kicking the trauma to the curb. I had learned a **lot** - about myself, about relationships, about psychology and how people tick. I had tamed many of my "triggers" and the symptoms had become more of a constant background noise. But they were still very much there. I had talked about them for ten years and they weren't going anywhere.

I decided I needed to try some new things. Here's a loosely organized timeline of my C-PTSD recovery journey:

Cognitive Behavioral Therapy - Also known as "Talk" therapy, this was my starting point. I spent over ten years with this same therapist and made some progress but I ended up feeling stuck in that progress for the last couple of years with him.

Essential Oils- This was my first foray into alternative therapies. My first shift with essential oils came when I opened up a bottle of a blend called "Trauma Life" and inhaled deeply. I immediately felt a shifting in my brain - as if a grip that had been holding it was releasing. I started to experiment with more and more essential oils and every one I tried continued to help my brain feel more free and release some of the gripping emotions. The nightmares settled down a bit, as did the flashbacks. My therapist began to notice a calmness and groundedness which he knew was not due to his efforts. He encouraged me to continue to work with the oils. The oils jump-started my recovery but were not the only tool I needed.

The Body Keeps the Score - I'm not sure what made me pick up Bessel Vanderkolk's book *The Body Keeps the Score* but this book became central to my full recovery. I suggest anyone on a recovery journey from PTSD read this book. This book shifted my understanding of PTSD from a condition of the mind to a condition of the brain and physiology. Reading this book was hard for me - it was as if Dr. Vanderkolk were writing a biography of my personal trauma experience. He seemed to understand my *body* intimately and what was going on within my skin, bones and organs. I finally understood why I couldn't talk my trauma away.

Dr. Peter Levine- About the same time I discovered Dr. Vanderkolk's book, I also stumbled across some videos (search on YouTube) created by Dr. Peter Levine where he demonstrates his work with war veterans. He was able to show in those videos how his work with clients actually helped them **physically** shift the trauma out of their bodies. He worked first to raise awareness of how the body experiences emotion and the fight/flight/freeze response and then helped his clients physically move their bodies to release that primitive trauma response. His book *Waking The Tiger* helped me put what I saw in those videos to work in my own body.

Emotional Freedom Techniques (aka as EFT or "Tapping") - After discovering the work of Levine and Vanderkolk, I began to search in earnest for body-based therapies I could teach myself.

On a chance visit to my chiropractor, we were talking about my trauma history and he had one of his office staff tap with me. She was inexperienced and naive, and that first tapping session was brief, emotionally painful, and left me triggered and dissociated for days afterwards. It was a horrible introduction to tapping for trauma!

However, I became curious about this body-involved technique which could arouse such strong feelings so quickly and I began to seek out everything I could find by its founder, Gary Craig. Eventually I would go through all his materials and then go on to become a certified Clinical EFT practitioner (Clinical EFT is what you need for trauma recovery! Watch out for amateurs who aren't prepared to handle the deep issues!).

Once I learned how to *properly* tap through my trauma history, I began to experience rapid recovery. I experimented with Tapping with essential oils and found I no longer needed the boost the oils gave me.

Movement Therapist - When essential oils and EFT began to help me take off on my recovery, I decided it was time to say goodbye to my beloved cognitive therapist. I turned to a beautiful soul of a woman - a dancer and therapist who labels her work "movement therapy." She helped me listen to the trauma signals my brain was sending to my body and locate areas of my body where I was physically holding on to my traumatic experiences. In the spirit of Peter Levine's Somatic Experiencing therapy, she helped me literally move the trauma out of my muscle memory and out of my body. In the six months I spent working with her, I accomplished more trauma recovery than I had in the 10+ years in Cognitive Therapy. She helped me gain a sense of agency over my own body and my own recovery process and taught me how to listen to and communicate with my *body's* distress signals. This was essential learning.

Qigong - This movement therapist introduced me to the Chinese yoga form Qigong (pronounced chee-gong if you've ever wondered!). This is a slow movement form which links breath to movement and is amazing for body awareness and feeling grounded and connected. Qigong has been central to creating positive daily habits and helping me feel safe in my own body. I continue learning this form.

Mindfulness Mentoring- At the same time I was gaining more and more skill with EFT, I was also meeting regularly with a mindfulness mentor. My mindfulness practice is now embedded into my daily life almost as naturally as breathing. The ability to stay present in each moment and not allow my thoughts to bang about in past regrets or future worries has been the underlying thread that has tied together all the other pieces of my recovery process.

This list represents the most used vehicles that moved me along in my journey out of C-PTSD. Along the way there have been other influencers who have clarified my understanding and helped me to teach others about their own relationship to the traumatic experiences in their lives - people such as Dan Siegel, Dawson Church, Lissa Rankin, and many others in the trauma research field.

If I had to point to any one part of this that I could not have recovered without, it would be understanding that my traumatic experiences themselves do not matter. Current trauma theory teaches that the brain always responds to threats to life and safety in the exact same way - and then embeds that response in the body. This is the central idea needed to build your own recovery toolbox.

Just as I listed what C-PTSD looked like for me, let me joyfully share what my recovered experience looks like:

- No more nightmares or flashbacks - ever
- Relaxed, connected time with friends in public places
- Responding to my children, husband and others out of love, kindness and thoughtfulness
- A visceral sense of grounding and peace from deep within myself
- Feeling present and connected to most situations
- Physically healthy
- Strong sense of agency and control over myself and situations in which I find myself

- Responding with curiosity and healthy detachment to new and old situations and emotions without judgement
- Willingness to accept responsibility for my actions and formulate a plan to change when needed
- Free from feelings of dread, doom, depression and shame
- Equipped with many different types of resources to use - and the determination to use them - whenever I begin to stray backwards on my path

Not everyone's journey will look the same. Some journeys take detours through addiction, or personality disorder, or physical illnesses, or co-dependent relationships or a myriad of other complications that require an extra layer of work and self-reflection. The key to beginning any Trauma Recovery journey is to begin with self-reflection about how your trauma has shaped the way your body responds to it.

The tools I used and listed here are the ones that I felt divinely led to explore and master. They were exactly what I needed in order to fully recover from the symptoms of C-PTSD. Your journey is bound to be equally as unique and varied. I share my journey to show that it can be done! You don't have to live like the person I described in the beginning of this post. You can live like the person I described at the end! Please, don't give up on yourself!

CLINICAL EFT BASIC "RECIPE"

MARY KALBACH
EMOTIONAL TRAUMA RECOVERY COACH

STEP ONE: RATE YOUR LEVEL OF ACTIVATION

Assign a number to the issue you wish to tap on. This number indicates how "activated" you are by this issue. If it is a physical pain a 0 would be no pain, a 10 would be the most pain possible.

For an emotional issue, a 0 might be "This issue is not at all affecting me and does not bother me" and a 10 might be "I can't think about this without feeling like I'm going to explode". Write down the number and where in your body you are feeling the effects of this issue.

STEP TWO: CREATE YOUR SET UP STATEMENT

Insert the name of your issue into the statement:

Even though I have this (name the specific issue), I deeply and completely accept myself and how I feel.

This helps you name your issue and accept it in the present moment

STEP THREE: TAP ON THE "KARATE CHOP" POINT

Tap continuously on the karate chop point on the side of your hand while you recite the Set Up Statement from step 2 three times.

The karate chop point is located on the fleshy part of the side of your hand below your pinky finger. It is ok to tap on either hand.

STEP FOUR: TAP ON THE REMAINING POINTS

Tap on each of the remaining points on the head, face, and torso about 7 times on each point.

You can tap with one hand on either side of the body or with both hands on both sides at once.

Recite your Reminder Phrase as you tap on these points.

STEP FIVE: BREATHE

Stop tapping, take a deep breath in, breathe out slowly, and focus your attention on the area of your body affected by your issue.

STEP SIX: RATE YOUR LEVEL OF ACTIVATION

Focus in on the part of your body affected by your issue and repeat Step One.

Compare this new number to the number you had when you started.

If you are not at a 0-1, repeat steps Two through Six until the issue is no longer causing a reaction in your body.

MARYKALBACH.COM @FOLLOWMARYKALBACH

MINDFUL MEDITATION

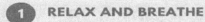

Feeling Heard, Seen and Understood

1 ### RELAX AND BREATHE

Find a comfortable, quiet place to sit. Breathe in deeply through your nose and out through your mouth. Try to pull the breath from your belly and imagine you can see your breath move through your body. Send it to all the parts of your body that are tired and tense and imagine relaxing each point of tension as it receives your breath.

2 ### BRING TO MIND A MEMORY

of a time when you felt seen, heard or understood. You may need to go way back in time or you may need to use your imagination and imagine someone who loves you telling you "I see you" or "I hear you" or "You're struggling so much. Let me help you".

3 ### NOTICE

the small details of that memory - did they smile at you? Give you a hug? Use a kind tone of voice? What words were said that made a positive impact on you? Put yourself back in that moment and notice everything about it.

4 ### TAKE IT IN

Does the memory bring up feelings somewhere in your body? Notice a warm feeling or a surge of pride in your gut or a yellow sensation in your chest - notice the pleasant feeling inside of you and imagine it growing and expanding and filling every part of your body from the top of your head to bottoms of your feet.

5 ### RELAX INTO THE FEELING

Take note of your breathing again. Let your breath spread the warmth of this feeling through your body on the inside. Relax into the feeling like sinking into a warm, bubbly bathtub. Let yourself feel immersed in the feeling of being heard, seen or understood all the way from deep inside you to the air around you.

6 ### TAKE A MENTAL PICTURE

of yourself in that bathtub so you can look at it whenever you need to. Imagine holding that picture up inside of you next to the feelings that arise the next time you feel unseen, unheard or misunderstood. Use the picture as a resource inside yourself that you can turn to whenever you need.

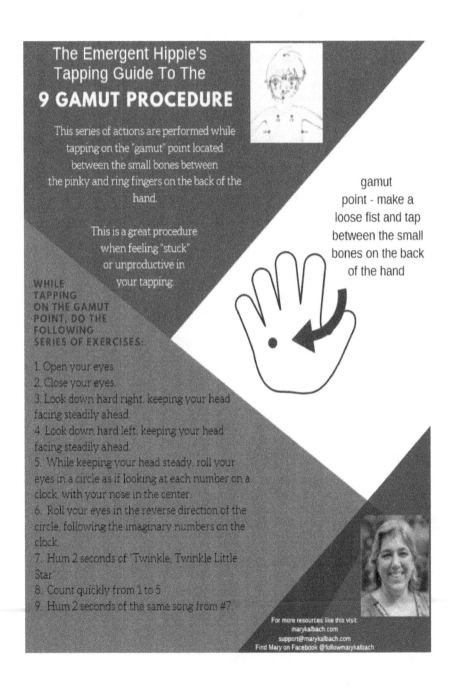

The Emergent Hippie's Tapping Guide To The
9 GAMUT PROCEDURE

This series of actions are performed while tapping on the "gamut" point located between the small bones between the pinky and ring fingers on the back of the hand.

This is a great procedure when feeling "stuck" or unproductive in your tapping.

gamut point - make a loose fist and tap between the small bones on the back of the hand

WHILE TAPPING ON THE GAMUT POINT, DO THE FOLLOWING SERIES OF EXERCISES:

1. Open your eyes
2. Close your eyes.
3. Look down hard right, keeping your head facing steadily ahead.
4. Look down hard left, keeping your head facing steadily ahead.
5. While keeping your head steady, roll your eyes in a circle as if looking at each number on a clock, with your nose in the center.
6. Roll your eyes in the reverse direction of the circle, following the imaginary numbers on the clock.
7. Hum 2 seconds of "Twinkle, Twinkle Little Star"
8. Count quickly from 1 to 5
9. Hum 2 seconds of the same song from #7.

For more resources like this visit:
marykalbach.com
support@marykalbach.com
Find Mary on Facebook @followmarykalbach

Author Spotlight
Mary Kalbach

Mary Kalbach holds degrees in Theater and Religious Studies. She has served her large, adoptive family as a therapeutic adoptive mom for over 20 years. She is certified as a Clinical EFT Practitioner by EFT Universe with a specialization in complex trauma. Mary is also a Certified Mindfulness Mentor by the Mindfulness Mentoring Institute and is currently working towards certification as a Psychodrama practitioner.

Mary serves on the Board of Directors for the Community for Holistic Integration, which seeks to integrate holistic health options throughout South Central Pennsylvania. She is a certified and insured Energy Psychology practitioner.

Mary teaches workshops and works with clients wherever her hippie soul dances.

Please contact Mary at support@marykalbach.com if you would like to work with her one on one or bring her to speak or workshop with your group or organization.

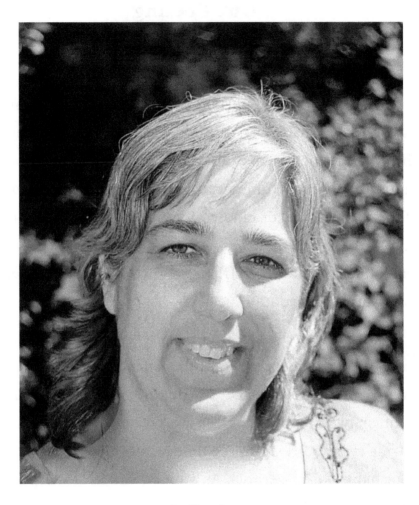

Learn more at marykalbach.com

Gut Feeling
Kerri Hample

I stood in the parking lot of a local restaurant with my fourteen-month-old son, sobbing. He had just thrown up his dinner all over me, the table, and the restaurant for the millionth time. We didn't go anywhere without a change of clothes for the whole family; and we only went places that were super family friendly, because it was almost certain that the end result would look similar to the current situation.

At every well visit, and by the way he was never well, the doctor would brush off our concerns. His entire body was covered in eczema; he wouldn't sleep more than an hour or two or at a time. He would arch his back in pain during every bottle from the time he was two weeks old. This poor baby was miserable. As a mom who is also a pediatric Occupational Therapist, I knew this wasn't right.

By the time my son was a year old, we tried eight different formulas, three medications for reflux, and a host of over the counter and prescription medications for his skin. Yet, he was still vomiting, regularly, still covered in eczema and still in pain most of the time!

I stood in the parking lot on the phone with the doctor and staring to the heavens begging God to help me, help me help him, and help this little boy be healthier so that he could be happy. The doctor did finally find medication that worked for his reflux and with that he did sleep, but he was just never well and always on edge. He threw up foods through preschool, kindergarten and first grade. He was allergy tested -- the only test patch that didn't react was the control. We began thinking allergy shots were going to be our ticket. Nope, sadly for him, they just made him sick. More colds, more ear infections and his eczema was at an all-time worst level.

With every visit to every specialist we inherited more prescriptions, more treatments; one would just cause new symptoms, requiring a new drug. At one point in our journey there was a gallon-sized Ziploc bag full of medications that he needed.

That bag was my breaking point. I knew my son couldn't spend his whole life on that many drugs and I knew he wasn't getting any better. I started doing my research and learned that we were far from alone --- lots of kids were having similar troubles. I came across the words "functional medicine" in my research when he was twelve. I was smitten. I couldn't get enough! Wow! I found doctors who wanted to find the root cause of chronic problems, to treat those problems with lifestyle changes instead of medications. It was music to my Occupational Therapy ears and especially my Mom heart.

I was so intrigued that I moved forward with a functional medicine health coaching certificate so that I could learn as much as I possibly could! And learn I did! While my son is not allergic to any foods, he is highly sensitive (IGA, not IGE) to dairy, gluten, soy, and wait for it... oats! The oatmeal lotion that the doctors had him bathing in for his eczema was one of his biggest triggers. All of the formulas that they switched him to, such as wheat and soy, he was sensitive to all of them! I had finally proven that I was not crazy, and that he really was in pain all of those years! So why didn't he just tell me that he was in pain?

As an Occupational Therapist, specializing in sensory processing, I have learned that in order to process pain, thirst, hunger, fatigue one must have intact interception. Most people think that we have five senses; true, we do. But we have three more! We have the external ones that everyone knows: sight (vision), smell (olfaction), taste (gustation), hearing (audition), and touch (somatosensation). We also have three internal: proprioception (tells us where our bodies are in space), vestibular (tells us how to correct our balance), and lastly interception (tells us how our body feels inside). Our bodies have receptors all over-- in our muscles, in our skin and in our gut.

The gut lining or microbiome is one sensitive system. Antibiotics and proton inhibitors (remember the infections and the reflux medications) destroy the good bacteria in the gut that keep the receptors happy. I always knew that even though my son has above average intelligence, and none of the markers for autism, he could not answer simple interception questions. For example, "Buddy, how does your body feel when you are full?" Answers that make sense would include "stomach is tight," "pants feel tighter," or "just know I don't need anymore." His answer is one that changed the course of my life.

"I know I'm full when my neck pulses." What? By now you know I am a researcher, so I needed to know more about this answer. So, like any other crazy mom trying to get the bottom of this to help her son, I started eating, and eating, eating. Yes, your neck does pulse. It's your vagal nerve right before you vomit! Like right before, you can barely stop it. Lightbulbs went off in my brain!

My journey to learn more about interception and food and how the gut dictates all has been a path I never sought; it found me! There is a pain like no other when a mom has cried all night, night after night because their child can't eat, sleep or poop without pain. Something happens to a mom when these things are challenging. Babies and kids eat five to seven times, sometimes more per day; they are supposed to sleep more than they are awake. I knew there was something that was just not right with my baby and yet no one would really listen or help.

Gastro-intestinal issues and kids with sleep, behavior and eating issues are commonplace. I believe with all my heart that kids do their best with what they have. I know that kids don't choose to misbehave, or cry all night, or run around the classroom. My journey, while it was not one I planned, has taught me how to help myself, my son, and so many others.

While I would not wish his first six years on anyone, I know all things have a purpose and he has taught me how to help others. Gut Feeling is my company where I help kids and their families eat well, so that they can feel well, so that they can do well. When kids eat well, they feel well; and when they feel well, they do their best!

My son is now fifteen, a healthy baseball player with big dreams. I used to think about his future and worry that he would be too sick to play, not anymore... five-ten, ripped, and ready to conquer his dreams --- including eating what he wants, when he wants and we both sleep instead of cry at night! I know we are not alone; I have met so many moms and kids with similar journeys! If you are looking for help to get started, I am more than happy to assist! Contact me at gutfeelingOT@gmail.com so that your kiddo can eat well, feel well, and at last, do well!

Author Spotlight

Kerri Hample

D r. Kerri Hample is an Occupational Therapist and Certified Functional Medicine Health Coach. She graduated from Thomas Jefferson University in 2000 with a Bachelor of Science in Occupational Therapy and graduated with a clinical doctorate in Occupational Therapy from Rocky Mountain University of Health Professions. In 2009 she completed both a certificate in health coaching from the Functional Medicine Health

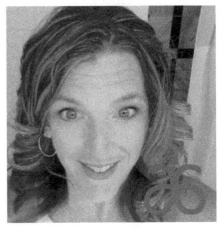

Coaching Academy and international certification. She is currently an Associate Professor of Occupational Therapy at Elizabethtown College and has a private health coaching practice where she is a Regional Vice President with Arbonne International. In her spare time, you can find her and her husband watching two awesome and amazing kids play baseball and compete in all start cheer.

717-361-1172   gutfeelingOT@gmail.com

Following The Stars
Angie Whitsel

I've always been fascinated by the stars. I was lucky to grow up in the woods, where there was no light pollution. Many nights were spent outside, blanket strewn across the soft grass, looking to the velvety sky adorned with twinkling lights. I even pestered my parents to let me go to Space Camp in fourth grade, but they said I would never utilize that knowledge in my life. How wrong they were!

My spiritual journey has been very ... eclectic. I have worked with energy and Spirit in so many different ways in the initial parts of my journey, but it wasn't until I took Reiki Sound, that I began to have a lot of a-ha moments about how energy truly works. I began to understand the rawest form of what creates energy- sound and vibration. If we think of The Big Bang, this is how it all started and why we are here!

I began to see an even deeper level of that age-old saying, "As Above, So Below. So Within, So Without." Human beings are most definitely the microcosm of the macrocosm. We really are stars wrapped in skin! For example, when a new star is born, it gives off a spark of light. When sperm meets an egg, it also gives off a flash of light. Some say this is the moment the soul arrives. Some say that planets are also beings ... angels ... gods and goddesses that carry their own energy signature and have their own consciousness. When a new star is born, is that flash of light the "soul" of the planet coming to life?

Or when stars split and divide into two, does this not replicate the division of cells? I could go on and on.

As I began to dig into this concept more, I realized that our auras are our own personal solar systems and our hearts are the Great Central Sun. I played around with this concept intuitively for a very long time and created my own version of "Celestial Reiki." Little did I know at the time that there was such a thing as Medical Astrology, a practice performed by ancient alchemical physicians.

Hippocrates has been quoted saying, "A physician without a knowledge of astrology has no right to call himself a physician." Astrology has changed my life. It has helped me to understand why we all act the way we do. It has given me a big-picture perspective and appreciation for the good, the bad, and the ugly of humanity. All personalities, in addition to all of our quirks, are for divine purpose. I absolutely believe we **chose** to be born into a specific energy of the zodiac in order to **experience** life in a way that helps us overcome lessons our souls need to grow to the next level of spiritual ascension.

To dive deeper, understand that not only do we take on the energy of our zodiac sign through personality traits, we also take on the health aspects of that sign as well. A well-balanced person usually does not have many issues. Unfortunately, due to modern living, less and less people are able to remain well balanced in body, mind, and soul. Many people take on the health issues of their zodiac sign and this is where the stars and healing meet. As a healer who loves the stars, I instantly fell in love with Medical Astrology. I realized how much astrology affects our health, how we hold our vital force energy, how our faces and bodies are formed, and how we are susceptible to different types of ailments and conditions under our individual Sun Signs.

How can one begin to understand Medical Astrology? I want to you to picture the typical circular astrology chart with the houses in order – Aries being first, with Pisces being last. Let's pretend that I take a scissors to that circle and cut it apart so that the circle falls into a straight line. Aries would be at the top and Pisces would be at the bottom. Now I want you to picture a human body standing beside this chart. Aries represents the head and Pisces represents the feet. It is imperative to understand that people born in different signs must be healed differently.

You do not need to be a Master Astrologer to do this work and some of the top Medical Astrology Masters will tell you this as well, but I do confess that the more you know about the stars, the better a physician you will be. I find myself back-tracking now, learning more astrology until I can move forward in my Medical Astrology practice. How would you feel about a surgeon who never took basic anatomy classes performing surgery on you or a loved one?

"What does a Medical Astrology healing session look like?" I am sure all practitioners work differently, but personally, I like to get the birth information of my client a week before I meet with them. This gives me ample time to plot and pull a very basic one-page natal birth chart. I then ask the client to fill out an "energy report" of their body and ask them to list all of their current health concerns and issues for comparison.

Medieval physicians would always treat the sun first and this is also where I begin. The sun was revered and was known to rule over the head and the heart, the two largest electric generators of the body. Remember, we are **electric** beings first and foremost! We must realize that we are beings of light, filled with and affected by energy. Our words are energy. Our thoughts our energy. Our emotions are energy. The food we eat is energy. When our energy is off, disease begins to fester within the body. This is why it is so important to mind your words and thoughts, eat raw and whole food diets, and address emotional and psychological issues. Once one energy center becomes unbalanced, if it is ignored for too long, it can begin to affect the other energy centers in your body and thus the downward spiral begins, affecting multiple organs and systems. This is usually the case, I have found, with autoimmune disorders in which modern medicine has a hard time diagnosing. So many times, there is unhealed trauma lying underneath that has been unaddressed.

Sitting with the client's chart, I determine what "zone" of the body their energy influences through their Sun Sign and what diseases this may bring up for the individual. I continue to dig for deeper meaning through what I like to call the "birth blueprint." Is their sun sign cardinal, fixed, or mutable? What "season" is their sign in? What element is their sun sign in? All of this matters in the beginning steps of Medical Astrology.

The elements play an enormous role in the vitality of each zodiac sign. For example, water signs tend to move their energy downwards, towards the feet. Water signs have the weakest vitality of the zodiac and a large part of this is because of how they hold their energy (or not hold onto it). Earth signs move their energy towards their center. This makes them the greatest "batteries" of the zodiac and they can sustain their energy over longer periods of time. Air signs tend to move their energy upwards, often making them feel ungrounded and "in the clouds." Fire signs move their energy outward and they use up their energy quickly, so they are likely to have a lot of energy at the beginning of the day but tend to burn out quickly because they expend their energy all at once.

In astrology, there are also three "health houses" that play a significant role in how we utilize our life force energy. By looking at planets in those houses, you may be able to see what else is adding its influence to the health equation. There are so many factors that go into diagnosing someone through Medical Astrology that I would take up this entire booklet. I hope that this gives you just a small taste of what Medical Astrology can show you. The following key points help us wrap up the diagnosis process into a nice little package.

Nine Key Points of Assessment

1)   The twelve signs compare to rulership of the body parts.

2)   Vitality and metabolism are measured through the Sun, Saturn and Mars.

3)   The distribution of the life force energy (or chi) is measured through the Moon.

4)   Overall body temperature is assessed through Saturn and Mars.

5)   Excess and deficiency are measured through the Lunar Modes.

6)   The bodily systems are measured through the planets in the signs and houses.

7)   The four elements measure how the vital force energy or chi if affected in each sign.

8)   The rate of flow of the vital force is measured through the three modes.

9)   Current time influences are measured through the transits and progressions.

Finally, what does healing look like in Medical Astrology? It is very much tied to both sound healing and alchemical processes. Sound and vibration mean everything when we commit to the "As Above, So Below" practice of this modality. I use tuning forks the most as they help me clear the biofield much easier because the tones help me pinpoint the anomalies in the aura through the sound waves of the different forks. I also use methods the ancient medieval physicians used – herbs, precious metals and alchemy. For example, I use gold to heal the heart, the Great Central Sun of the body. Gold has been revered by the ancients as the ultimate healing metal and was made into elixirs and worshipped. Much like how some of us drink monatomic gold today, there are many benefits to certain metals in balancing the body.

Following my heart into the stars has brought a wealth of discovery, both of the self and of all the energy with which we interact in the world. As a young girl gazing up at the stars, I had dreamed of connecting to the celestial presence sensed, and by healing through Medical Astrology, I now recognize that I am and have always been a luminescent part.

Author Spotlight
Angie Whitsel

Angie Whitsel provides a variety of holistic and alternative healing services and classes both in person and via internet. Reiki, Starseeds, Oracle and Tarot Readings and much more. Her knowledge of Medical Astrology, in combination with her intuition, genuine desire to assist, and authentic nature make her an excellent support on your healing journey.

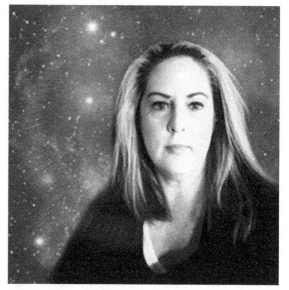

717-884-2192

https://www.AngieWhitsel.com

www.facebook.com/AngieWhitsel

www.youtube.com/StarsSpiritHealing

A Simple Shift
Kimber Bowers

A tear falls expanding into a tiny imperfection on the crisp white sheet, just as all the perceived failures, the should haves, the could haves, of my miserably long young life spill out to taint the open canvas of this very moment... My mind weaves a million different worst-case scenarios. My body slumps under the weight of negative expectation and perceived loss. Pulling the covers over my head, I don't want to move. I want to stay snuggled in the security of soft warm blankets and the safety of solitude. I am *tired*. I am tired from the heartache, tired from the struggling, tired from the unmet expectations, tired from all the running that doesn't seem to get me anywhere.

Have you been here? Have you felt this?

Unwilling to face another day, certain that I cannot take another moment, I burrow into the soft caress of my bed, refusing to open my eyes to the light – refusing to let that light in. I cannot bear another disappointment. I cannot risk another broken heart. There are jobs to do, demands to meet, and chores accruing that I just don't have the energy for. There are illnesses to manage, expectations to fall short of, losses to bear, and bills to pay. There are disappointments to feel, pain to manage, and complaints to hear and I'm not sure I'm up for it. There are dishes to wash and people to take care of, and I'm not even sure that I know how. I just don't *feel* like it... *any* of it...

"Wake up!" I hear my husband urge.

"I'm awake," I mutter as I pull the covers higher waiting for him to go away... wanting it all to just go *away*.

But there are also people, he reminds me softly, people whom I love... and like a splinter in the darkness, that awareness expands.

There are smiles to share, hands to hold, and hugs to embrace. There are pets to snuggle, growth to witness, flowers to smell, breezes to feel, seeds to plant, and adventures to take. There are games to play, music to hear, art to create, beauty to see, and touches to accept – touches that go so deep I cannot imagine never to have felt them. There are experiences for which I would not trade a single moment of my pain. There are connections for which I would live that pain a million times over in exchange. There are insights of grace and joy so rich that they are worth the risk, moments that might never have happened without surviving the breaks.

"You're not awake until your feet hit the floor," I hear my Pappy direct from beyond the grave and a sigh of deep knowing escapes my lips.

Light cannot get in until I open to it. All the stressors become doorways to deeper experience. Every shadow becomes a window to light. Every loss becomes space for new gain. Every failure becomes a steppingstone to this very moment, if I but can make that simple shift.

Every moment has the power to bring connection, wholeness, and growth (even the hard ones). Am I willing to step into this gift? Am I able to shift my focus to it?

The covers come down. My weight shifts. Pushing to the bed's edge, I gingerly place my feet upon the floor. Focusing on this one moment and trusting in the growth that it contains, *I open.* Seeing the beauty of the highs and lows without needing to control it, this day will unfurl as divinely intended. Standing, I let light in, open to whatever blessing this moment brings. However guised it may be, I trust in it– *open to receive.*

In each breath lies a **choice**...
A choice to bring the spiritual being into physical
expression
A choice to allow the flow of soul through skin...
through hand... through touch... through life... through
action

A choice to bring these two worlds (being and doing,

faith and action) together

In a beautiful collision that changes everything.

Such a simple movement...

The inhale and exhale of breath over lips...

Carrying Divine presence into the world...

If only we are willing to focus on the opportunity

Each breath brings in.

On what are you focusing?

Meditation for Acceptance

Kimber Bowers

S it comfortably anywhere that you like
and focus on your breath.
Allow awareness of your breath to expand.

Notice the temperature and sensation of the air moving up
through the nasal passages and down into your
diaphragm... Allowing it to expand.

Follow the rise and fall allowing the rhythm to relax you
even more.

Enhance your willingness to accept and **be** in this
moment, by tuning into the vibration of it

Expand your awareness from your breathing to any
sensations you feel in your body – all the way into the feel
of your heart beating, the release of tension in your
muscles, any internal sensations, and all the way out to
the temperature of air on your skin, the feel of the clothes
on your body, the way your weight distributes on whatever
you are sitting against...

Allow yourself to fully feel and experience where you are
right now.

Expand your awareness now to any sounds –
all the way into the sound of your heart beating,
the sound of your swallow, the sound of your breath,
out to the sounds in the world around you,

the tick of the clock, the hum of an appliance,
vehicles or animals or winds outside --
allowing yourself to hear all of the sounds
and accepting them all as a part of the rhythm of *now*,
all working together to bring you the peace an beauty of
this moment.

I am whole. I am connected. I am rooted in the **now** –
open to the rhythm, to the beauty, to the magical vibration
of all that is currently here for me.
Able to easily separate that which is passing
from that which is eternal –
my own wholeness, my own connection, my own love, my
own peace.

Stepping away from the need to decipher and allowing my
growth through just **be**ing with it.

- Listen to an enhanced guided version of this meditation for free at www.lovinglighthw.com/downloads
- Previously published in Kimber Bowers, *Awaken Your Joy: A Practical Guide to Embrace Fulfillment.* (P.A.V.E. Press, 2019). 40.
- Copies available at mybook.to/AwakenYourJoy

Author Spotlight

Kimber Bowers

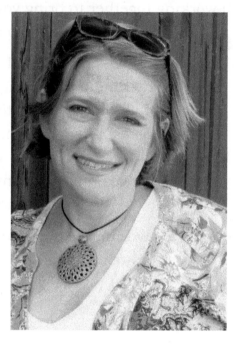

Rev. Kimber Bowers, CCHt is an Amazon Bestselling Author, fun-loving mom, artist, nature enthusiast, and Integrative Mind Body Wellness Practitioner in Dallastown, PA.

As an empath who suffered most of her life with Clinical Depression and Anxiety, she has now discovered the keys to joy and fulfillment and has made it her mission to help you find yours! When she is not busy guiding others to discover the Love that **is**, you will find her getting creative, hiking with the kids, or foraging for the essence of wildflowers in the grass.

Read about her online course helping you create and integrate the shifts necessary to embrace a life of fulfillment at www.lovinglighthw.com/open-receive

Check out her books at bit.ly/KimberBowers

Loving Light Holistic Wellness, Dallastown, PA

www.lovinglighthw.com   (410) 241-2635

Resilience
Denise VanBriggle

23 April 1977

by Jimmy Santiago Baca

It seems
prison confines and destroys—
it does, I know, no need to argue
the point, just look at these
infamous edifices thrashing out,
consuming
human beings like bait sardines,
but I cannot stand on this.
Yes, the great iron hand of prison
crushes all in its grasp,
the mind and soul become
feeble sacks
filled with rotten fruits,
a gunnysack crumpled in a dark cell.
but to control your mind and soul
is to become a stronger hand,
embanking gently the loose clods
of ravaged and confused past
so the river of your heart
and clear streams of your soul
may pass,
full and freely, into rich fallow beds
of freedom, waiting for you
even in prison,

even in prison; many will not understand this,
but I will say that we can
overcome,
not today, tomorrow, or next month,
but at the very moment
one decides upon it.

Baca, J. (2001). *A Place to Stand* New York, Grove
Press.

In March of 2005 my daughter Erika lay in a hospital bed recuperating from serious lung surgery not long after the birth of her first child, and my first grandchild. At Christmastime I had just adopted a cell dog from a Virginia prison and had started a friendly correspondence with the inmate who trained my Izzygirl, a gorgeous Australian Shepherd mix. A concerned friend gave me a copy of Baca's memoir *A Place to Stand* with the firm directive, "This book is a must read for anyone associated with the prison system in any way." Books have always been my go-to form of escape, so I thought reading might calm my fears as I sat steady watch over my firstborn, now the ripe old age of twenty-seven. This particular poem triggered a heart-opening, body-shaking cry, and I vowed to meet the man whose words evoked such a powerful release. You see, on 23 April 1977 while Baca penned the poem from his Arizona prison cell, I lay in a hospital bed in Harrisburg, just a few floors away, cradling the then three-day-old Erika whose unlikely prison had been her own mother's womb. (Who knew these wide hips of mine housed a pelvis too small to allow for safe passage through the birth canal?) After a 24-hour struggle, the doctor was forced to cut her free. My beautiful baby girl entered the world full of light and love and possibility. At that moment, I had no idea what trials and tribulations her future would hold.

Between 2008 and 2011, Erika endured another scary lung surgery and two high-risk pregnancies—both requiring post-delivery surgeries--yet today I am blessed to enjoy not one but three healthy grandchildren. In 2008, as another literary diversion, I read Elizabeth Gilbert's *Eat, Pray, Love* and was inspired to travel to Italy. Not long after I returned home, I had the opportunity to meet Jimmy Santiago Baca who re-kindled my internal social justice fire. He has become friend, mentor, and muse. Together, Gilbert and Baca re-ignited my love of writing. I currently serve as an Official Visitor of the Pennsylvania Prison Society and recently co-authored a collection of poetry and curricular ideas titled *Feeding the Roots of Self-Expression and Freedom* with Jimmy Santiago Baca and Kym Sheehan (Teachers College Press, 2018).

Through their daily resilience and courage, Erika Dupes, Jimmy Santiago Baca, and Elizabeth Gilbert model passionate, compassionate, and purposeful living. With their lives as models, I have learned to set fear aside and nudge myself into public spaces and places of vulnerability. I did it, and you can, too. Be brave. Be fearless. Decide in this moment.

Author Spotlight
Denise VanBriggle

Denise VanBriggle is a writer, Reiki Master Teacher, Certified Crystal Healer, ReikiVoice and ReikiSound Practitioner, and Transformational Reiki Practitioner. Prior to her retirement, she was a career educator, former director of the Capital Area Writing Project at Penn State University, and a Teacher-Consultant with the National Writing Project.

Since her retirement in 2011, after 34 years of service Kindergarten through university, she honors her healing gifts and fuels her love of teaching and writing through her small business located in Suite A - Brownstone Station, Hummelstown, PA.

Denise spends most days following her combined passions as she explores the power of the expressive arts to act as change agents, perspective shifters, and resilience builders in her own life and the lives of others.

Her first book, *Feeding the Roots of Self-Expression and Freedom* (with acclaimed poet Jimmy Santiago Baca and teacher-poet Kym Sheehan) is a compendium of curricular ideas and probing questions designed to complement Baca's early prison poems and the documentary film, *A Place to Stand,* based on Baca's memoir of the same title.

Her second collection, *Erato*, is on tap for publication in the spring of 2020. For more information, visit www.denisevanbriggle.com

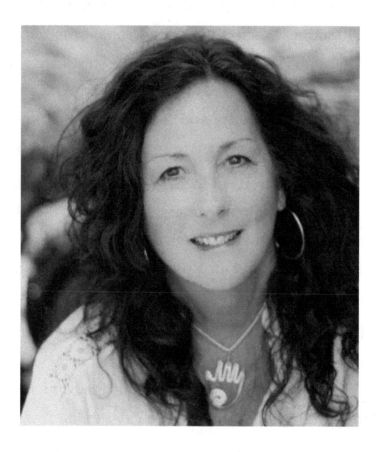

The Lotus Eater
Michele Lefler

My parents divorced when I was four. My father had custody of my two sisters and me. This was almost unheard of in the early 1980s. I believe that this has shaped my life more than anything else. I was at a critical stage in life where their divorce affected me more than my sisters. My older sister was nine and had spent the critical early years with both parents. At two, my younger sister was young enough that she could adjust to a change in parentage easier. I was at a stage where I knew what was going on and internalized it more. I became a people pleaser, and that led to a serious case of perfectionism and obsessive-compulsive disorder.

I believe that my weight issues also stem from my parents' divorce. A lack of knowing I was loved unconditionally led me at a very young age to use food as a way to self soothe and comfort. I know I have been surrounded by family who loved me but knowing it in your head is not the same as knowing it in your heart. And that's even more true when you're four. I also believe that this constant life-long struggle with my weight led, in part, to my perfectionism. I have never been able to control my weight and my body. But, I'd be damned sure to control everything else in my life.

I have always struggled with the need for everyone to approve of me. In my mind approval equaled love. As a result, I have often made choices and decisions that were not authentic to me, but were made out of a desire to win someone else's love. The earliest instance of this that I can remember occurred in my teens. I began exploring witchcraft and new age spirituality. I read books and explored whatever way I could without drawing a lot of attention to what I was doing. When my family found out I was chastised and told I needed to repent and come back to Jesus so that I wouldn't die and spend eternity in Hell. So, I did.

When I was in Kindergarten, I decided I wanted to be a teacher. I quickly realized that my good grades made my teachers and family happy so I thought it would really make them happy if I grew up to be a teacher. Most children change career aspirations often. I did not. When my family showed happiness at the fact that I loved school and wanted to be a teacher it became my lifelong mission. I never questioned that desire. I graduated high school, went to college for the teacher education program, and discovered I didn't really like the idea of being a teacher. I finished the program, though, but didn't become a teacher when I graduated. Twelve years later, however, I did. I hated it. After three years I left that field for another.

I have struggled with relationships trying to find love and making some poor decisions. Not all of my romantic relationships were poor choices, but some were. After my junior year of college, I met a man and started dating him. We quickly fell in love and became quite serious. When I went back for my senior year, he visited me every other weekend- making the four-hour drive to spend a few days with me. After my graduation I returned home, and we fell into a routine. I soon wanted more from our relationship, but he wasn't ready. He ended our relationship after two years. I was devastated.

A few months after this relationship ended, I met another man. Two weeks later I married him. Of course, this marriage didn't last. When the novelty of our marriage wore off, he started to show his true colors. He had several affairs. I forgave him. His gaslighting took a new turn when he decided he no longer wanted to be married to me. Instead of leaving he wanted to blacken my name and tarnish my reputation. He, of course, denied his affairs and tried to arrange for me to sleep with someone else. I didn't, but he told all of our friends that I did, anyway. I quickly found out who my friends were. After two years, at age 25, we divorced.

Two years later I met and married my second husband. We lived a decent life together. We loved each other with a passion. He struggled with mental illness, however, and that placed a major strain on our marriage. We did everything we could to work through it and did as well as could be expected. In May 2011, I came home from work and found that he had passed away.

After the initial phases of grief, I started to look at my life. I began to have little doubts about my Christian faith. I began to ask myself questions. It wasn't long after that until I decided that I really wanted to ask these questions. The faith I grew up with was not welcoming of these questions. I began to look elsewhere. I had always felt a special connection to Judaism, so I turned there. I began reading everything I could about Judaism and gravitating more and more toward it as a culture and religion. It wasn't a linear path, but in 2016, I completed my conversion to Judaism when I sat before the beit dein and entered the mikveh.

The conversion process included choosing my Jewish name. I chose the name Chaya Levana which means Living Moon. Chaya represents that I am finally living my authentic life. It also represents that I am, quite literally, still living. I chose to add the name Levana to honor the moon. I have always loved the moon. Its feminine energy speaks to me, and the moon has special significance for Jewish women.

Over the past several years I have added holistic therapies to my life to help me heal emotionally. This has helped me in ways that nothing else has. Meditation and Reiki are a balm to my soul. The self-inflicted wounds brought on by perfectionism have scabbed over and are healing. I no longer feel like a raw mess. They have given me the strength to look at myself and ask deep questions. I have become a stronger woman, no longer content to live my life based on other people's ideas of what is best for me.

I have further embraced the fact that Judaism not only allows questions but encourages it. Jews are known as the people of the book for a reason, and it extends beyond the literal meaning of our holy book. We read, study, ask questions, and learn. I have added many aspects of Buddhism into my walk as well as Celtic spirituality to honor my Scottish heritage. I also infuse a lot of earth based, hoodoo and conjure into my walk as well. I am becoming more and more vocal in my political beliefs, and those are fully fused with my spiritual beliefs as well. Feminism has been a huge recent influence on my spirituality.

The tools I have used to heal myself — meditation, Reiki, and blended spirituality- have become like an intoxicant for me. They have changed me, and I don't want to go back to the life I had before. They are like a lotus in my life.

The lotus is a symbol of beauty surrounded by ugliness. It is a sacred symbol in Buddhism, Hinduism, and ancient Egyptian religion. Known for its supreme beauty, it symbolizes purity, rebirth, transformation, and spiritual enlightenment. The lotus grows in murky water and opens into a beautiful clean flower. The juxtaposition of the flower next to the mud from which it grows has leant to the mystic and spiritual meaning behind the plant.

Imagine that you are standing next to a pond. The water is dark and muddy. You try to see the bottom but all you can see is the silt floating around in the water. You also see a flower. It is breathtaking in all of its exquisiteness. The light pink teardrop petals are clustered around a bright yellow center. The petals look like fingers on a hand cupped to hold the center. The entire blossom sits on a dark green pad floating on top of the muddy water. This is the lotus. If you wade through the muddy water and get close enough you can see that the "perfect" flower has blemishes. But they aren't noticeable. Even if you did see them, they don't matter for the flower is so beautiful against the mud that it doesn't matter. The mud doesn't take away from the flower. The lotus enhances the mud.

We find the idea of the lotus as transformational in Greek mythology. The ancient poet Homer related the tales of the lotus eaters in *The Odyssey*. Odysseus and his men were returning from Troy when a storm raged and blew them off course to an unknown island. Odysseus sent his scouts to the island. They encountered a people who survived off eating the native lotus. The inhabitants of this island gave the plant to Odysseus' scouts. When they ate it they became blissful, sleepy, and unaware of their normal duties. When his scouts failed to return to the ship, Odysseus sent out more scouts. They also failed to return. Odysseus ended up going to the island himself in search of his men. The locals offered him the plants to eat, but Odysseus refused. He found his men who were unwilling to return to the ship, Odysseus had to drag them back and put them in chains or they would not have returned.

Alfred, Lord Tennyson brought Homer's story to a modern age when he wrote his poem, *The Lotos-Eaters* in 1832. In the chorus, Odysseus' men have eaten the lotus and are now seeing the world around them through the eyes of their inner peace. They no longer want to return to Ithaca and the life they led before eating the lotus. They will remember their old lives, but they have no desire to go back. They are content with eating the lotus.

Like Odysseus's men, I have eaten the lotus and it has changed my life. Unlike his men, however, I am not content to lie still. I do not want to go back, but I want to share the lotus with others. I know how meditation and energy medicine have transformed my life. I see that I am a better person. I cannot be selfish and keep this to myself. My desire now is to introduce others to the life changing magic of eating the lotus.

My name is Chaya Levana. I am a Lotus Eater.

Communing With Ancestors Meditation
Michele Lefler

B egin by finding a comfortable position. (Pause) I recommend lying in savasana (corpse pose) flat on your back. Arms by your side with palms facing up. Legs straight on the floor. (Pause) If this is uncomfortable for you, please feel free to bend your knees with your feet flat on the floor. (Pause) If you prefer to sit, assume a comfortable position with your hands on your lap and your palms facing up. (Pause).

Now, close your eyes and take a deep breath and exhale. (Pause). Breathe normally for a bit. (Pause). Don't try to force your breath. Just breathe as you normally would. (Pause). In (pause) and out. (Pause). In (pause) and out. (Pause.) Now, watch yourself breathing. Notice how your chest and belly move with the inhalation. (Pause). And now notice the movement of your exhalation. (Pause). Keep breathing as you normally would and notice how your body moves with each breath (Long pause).

On the next inhale, tighten the muscles in your face. Hold the breath for a moment, and then relax your face as you slowly exhale. (Pause). Do the same with your shoulders. Tighten your shoulder muscles as you inhale. (Pause). Now, slowly exhale and release your shoulder muscles. (Pause). Inhale deeply, tightening the chest muscles. (Pause). And slowly exhale releasing the tension in your chest. Continue with your belly. Tighten your belly as you breathe in. Hold (pause) and release as you exhale. Breathe in and tighten your buttocks. (Pause) And now, release. Breathe in, stretching your legs. (Pause). And now exhale and release. Tighten your feet and toes as you breathe in. (Pause) And release.

Continue breathing your normal breath. (Pause). Just be aware of the gentle inhale and exhale. (Long pause.)

Visualize yourself outside standing at the beginning of a path. (Pause). The sky above you is blue and the clouds are fluffy like cotton balls. You notice that there is no one or nothing around you. There is only a path before you and a vast expanse behind you. (Pause.) You look into the distance and see a smudge of darkness on the horizon. You don't know what it is, but you want to find out.

You begin walking along the path towards the smudge. (Long pause.) After a few moments you realize that you are not alone. An animal is with you. You don't know where the animal came from, but you know that it is there to guide you. (Pause.) Reach down and touch the animal. Feel its fur if it has fur. This animal may be scaly, or it might be slimy. Spend a few moments communing with the animal before continuing along the path. (Long pause.)

You begin walking again, and before you realize it, the dark smudge on the horizon has taken shape into a large forest before you. You are almost there. (Pause.) Once you reach the forest you are curious about what is inside. Your animal guide has already darted into the forest, and you decide to follow.

There are smooth rocks along the path now, but you are easily able to tread over and around them. At the edge of the forest there are saplings growing on each side of the path. The saplings soon give way to large towering trees. There are so many trees around you. There are all different kinds of trees. Some trees are tall, and some are short. Some trees have rough bark, while others are smooth. You look around you and notice all the different types of trees.

As you continue walking the path begins to slope gently upward. You feel the breeze as it blows around you, its gentle fingers enveloping you in the soft coolness. You pause for a moment to enjoy the breeze. As you breathe deeply you inhale the earthy forest scent around you. You take several more deep breaths trying to pinpoint the different smells- soil, trees, moss, dirt. (Pause.)

You hear the sounds around you. Birds are twittering as they fly above. Twigs are snapping and leaves are crunching as woodland animals go about their day. They are hiding from sight, but still going about with whatever they need to do this day.

You begin walking again, and notice that your animal guide has not left your side. Continue walking forward and upward, enjoying the forest around you. (Long pause.)

You reach an opening in the forest. You are standing outside a large stone circle. There are twelve stones and inside you notice a single tree. This tree is much thicker around the trunk than the other trees in the forest. You notice that the trunk is gnarled and the branches are heavy. You can tell that this tree is old. You follow your animal guide through the stones and to the tree. Now you can see that there is an opening in the tree trunk. You reach out to feel the bark when your animal guide enters the tree. You follow.

There are steps inside the tree. They are carved into the dirt and are covered with lush green moss. They lead down into the earth. You follow your animal guide deeper and deeper into the earth under this tree. You notice the gnarled roots twisting and turning into knots. You see the roots have curved round and round into geometric shapes, knotting in and out of each other. It is dark inside the tree, but when you reach the bottom you can see a flickering light ahead. You walk down a narrow hallway toward the light and realize it is coming from numerous candles inside an opening.

As you reach the end of the hallway your animal guide darts inside a room. You follow and enter a cozy round room illuminated by many candles. The walls are smooth packed earth, and the floor is smooth with a little dirt. You can see roots in the dirt walls and floor, but the dirt has been packed tight around them.

There are also people inside this room. When you enter, the people look toward you and they all begin smiling. These people range in age from young to very old. There are both men and women. You notice they all have similar features and realize they must be related somehow.

An ancient woman with gray hair and a wizened face stands and walks toward you. She tells you that this is your family tree and that everyone gathered in this room below the tree are your ancestors. You sigh deeply and realize you had been holding your breath. The old woman puts her arm around you and invites you to sit with your ancestors. She promises that they have many stories to tell you. You join her on the floor, and everyone surrounds you. You start to introduce yourself and then realize they already know exactly who you are. You melt into the warmth of their embrace and listen to the wisdom they have to share.

(Long Pause- several minutes — length to meet your desire.)

After a while you realize that it is time to begin the journey back to your own time and place. You thank your ancestors for their wisdom and promise to return to speak with them again another time. You leave the room and go back down the hallway. You reach the moss-covered stairs and climb back up through the tree roots. You exit the tree and walk back out of the stone circle. You look back and smile at your family tree knowing you will, indeed, return to this place. You make your way back through the forest and out on the path. The sun has descended, and the moon is out. You notice the twinkling stars as you walk back to where you started.

(Pause.)

When you are ready you may open your eyes. Take a few moments to reflect on the wisdom your ancestors shared with you.

Note: You may wish to journal after this meditation to remember what your ancestors shared with you.

Author Spotlight
Michele Lefler

Michele Lefler is a certified holistic healer, Gendai Reiki Master, and certified life coach. Her experience in meditation, spiritual studies, and coping with grief anchor her work with clients. Michele is currently working on her first novel which she hopes to have finished in the near future. Michele lives in south central Pennsylvania with her husband, dog, and two turtles. She enjoys traveling and visiting historic sites.

To join her mailing list, receive her ebook On Hermetics, and/or learn about special offers and upcoming writing projects, visit her website, livingmoonmeditation.com

Connect with Michele
> FB: livingmoonmeditation
> TW: livingmoonmed
> IG: livingmoonmeditation

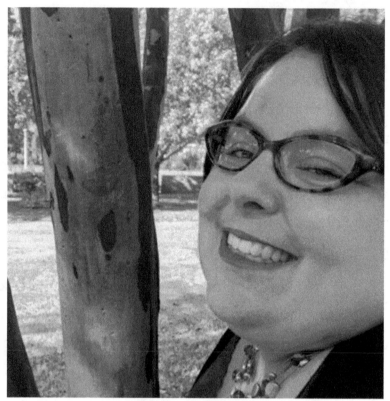

Michele Llefler

Living Moon Meditations

Collective Communication Empowers
Erec Smith

I am a professor of rhetoric studies, which, most simply, can be defined as the study of effective communication. Based on common trends in interpersonal communication across various aisles—political, cultural, religious, etc.—one could assume that my job is more important now than it ever has been in our society's history. However, to move from the study of communication to the remedy for miscommunication is not a small step. In order to accomplish the latter, one may have to look into the psychological and even spiritual realms of humanity.

Recently, I have come to realize that the basis of miscommunication can be understood as a general sense of disempowerment. That is, many do not feel truly empowered and, in an attempt to cope with this, resort to defensiveness, close-mindedness, and insularity to protect themselves from outside forces. This is to say that many people lack what Psychologist George Kohlrieser calls a "secure base," which he defines as "a person, place, goal or object that provides a sense of protection, safety and caring and offers a source of inspiration and energy for daring, exploration, risk taking and seeking challenge."[1]

It may be the case that if a person lacks a sufficient secure base, many endeavors taken, including the simple endeavor of communication with others, is really a veiled attempt to acquire or protect a secure base. When this happens, disagreement is seen as an attack, differing views of others are seen as indictments on one's own views, and differing lifestyles are seen as existential threats. Feelings of disempowerment and a lack of a secure base may be the biggest obstacles for effective and civil communication.

So, what can be done about this? Well, the first step toward gaining a sense of empowerment is to have a clear understanding of what it is. Definitions of empowerment abound, but for our purposes I believe that the definition derived from empowerment theory could be most beneficial. According to psychologist Marc Zimmerman, empowerment is "a process by which people, organizations, and communities gain mastery over issues of concern to them."[2] Perhaps most importantly, empowerment starts at the "individual level of analysis."[3] This last description is worth emphasizing. Empowerment starts with the individual and, ideally, grows into collective experience and collective

---

1. George Kohlrieser, *Care to Dare: Unleashing Astonishing Potential Through Secure Base Leadership* (San Francisco, CA: Jossey-Bass, 2012).
2-3. Marc Zimmerman, "Psychological Empowerment: Issues and Illustrations," *American Journal of Community Psychology*, 23.5 (1995), 581

action that "includes active engagement in one's community and an understanding of one's sociopolitical environment."[4]

A full exploration of this theory of empowerment is too large for the scope of this short essay, but we can touch on the importance of individuality and personal responsibility when it comes to empowerment. So, I have decided to focus on the concept of Positive Outlook, a component of emotional intelligence imperative to personal empowerment. Let's go with psychologist Daniel Goleman's definition.

> Positive Outlook is the ability to see the positive in people, situations, and events. It means persistence in pursuing goals, despite setbacks and obstacles. You can see the opportunity in situations where others would see a setback that would be devastating, at least for them. You expect the best from other people. It's that glass-half-full outlook that leads you to believe that changes in the future will be for the better.[5]

This definition may induce eye rolls from people who recognize such statements as "pie in the sky" thinking. The

---

4. Marc Zimmerman, "Psychological Empowerment: Issues and Illustrations," *American Journal of Community Psychology,* 23.5 (1995), 582
5. Daniel Goleman, "Positive Outlook: An Introduction," in *Positive Outlook: A Primer* (Florence, MA: More Than Sound, 2017), Loc 114.

concept of Positive Outlook may be interpreted as a belief that people who are truly victimized in society only need to think positively for their lives to change. This is not necessarily the case. Those with a strong grasp of Positive Outlook know to stave off *knee-jerk* negative reactions to a situation. Thus, Positive Outlook can enhance communication because the undesired actions of others are not automatically labeled negative. This is not to say that those behaving badly would be let off the hook; it is to say that necessary conversations are more likely to take place instead of an automatic shunning of an alleged culprit.

Again, the Positive Outlook competency is often mistaken as a synonym for wishful thinking. In addressing this tendency, Goleman shows that Positive Outlook is more aligned with the self-efficacy and positive self-regard. A pessimistic outlook attributes negative outcomes to personal failings or inevitably negative circumstances. People with an optimistic outlook recognize that negative outcomes are setbacks, challenges, and even opportunities for growth. Goleman calls the purposeful selection of the positive "dispositional optimism,"[6] which denotes the willingness to achieve goals one values and sees as realistic. Goleman writes that "rather than advocating for an 'optimistic under all circumstances' perspective, what

---

6. Daniel Goleman, "Positive Outlook: An Introduction," in *Positive Outlook: A Primer* (Florence, MA: More Than Sound, 2017), Loc 227

might be most effective is cultivating a generally optimistic outlook that is tempered by realistic pessimism."[7] This concept distinguishes Positive Outlook from wishful thinking or an unrealistic take on things.

Here is where rhetorician Kenneth Burke's concept of the "terministic screen" comes into play. According to Burke, the way we speak about things directs attention to some things and not others. All sincere language use is a reflection of reality, but "[e]ven if any given terminology is a *reflection* of reality, by its very nature as a terminology it must be a *selection* of reality; and to this extent it must function also as a *deflection* of reality."[8] Burke continues, "Here the kind of deflection I have in mind concerns simply the fact that any nomenclature necessarily directs the attention into some channels rather than others."[9] Positive Outlook, then, is a recognition of the arbitrary nature of these selections and deflections when reflecting on reality. A positive outlook may prompt the deflection of defeatist thinking and a selection of optimistic thought that can better see the positive potential in a situation.

The tendency to consistently select the negative over the positive, what many psychologists call negative emotionality, is a key component in failed communication.

---

7. Daniel Goleman, "Positive Outlook: An Introduction," Loc 248

8-9. Kenneth Burke, *Language as Symbolic Action*, in *The Rhetorical Tradition: Readings From Classical Time to the Present* 2nd Ed, Edited by Patricia Bizzell and Bruce Herzberg (New York: Bedford St. Martin's Press, 2001), 1341

Psychologist Scott O. Lilienfeld defines negative emotionality (NE) as "a pervasive temperamental disposition to experience aversive emotions of many kinds, including anxiety, worry, moodiness, guilt, shame, hostility, irritability, and perceived victimization."[10] Citing studies spanning twenty-five years, Lilienfeld continues to write, "[i]ndividuals with elevated levels of NE tend to be critical and judgmental of both themselves and others, vulnerable to distress and emotional maladjustment, and inclined to focus on the negative aspects of life... They also tend to be vigilant and overreactive to potential stressors"[11] and are "prone to interpreting ambiguous stimuli in a negative light."[12] Could negative emotionality be both the cause and effect in ineffective and/or uncivil communication? Perhaps.

Of course, I want to be clear that I am not shaming people with mental conditions that result in intense feelings of anxiety or those suffering from traumatic experiences. Getting over such things is easier said than done. I am, however, pointing out that, quite often, negative outlooks are a result of our curation of experiences. The same occurrence can be experienced much differently if seen from a positive disposition as opposed to a negative one. An occurrence can look vastly different depending on whether

---

10-12. Scott O. Lilienfeld, "Microaggression: Strong Claims, Inadequate Evidence." *Perspectives on Psychological Science* 12.1 (2017): 163

it is experienced from a secure base or an insecure base. I believe that acknowledging the concepts of terministic screens and Positive Outlook can help us be more cognitive of our dispositions, our selections and deflections. Thus, such acknowledgement can go a long way in improving how we communicate with one another.

This does have a spiritual component to it. One can see the confluence Positive Outlook and terministic screens as a wordy version of the maxim "energy goes where attention flows," or the common idea among spiritual leaders that we create our own reality. Well, it is, but couching this idea in theories of rhetoric and empowerment may help us focus on how our attention in communication can enhance interpersonal relations and promote civility. One can notice one's tacit seeking of a secure base, one's arbitrary selection of the negative, and work to see the positive in an interaction, even one that involves a truly hostile person. Of course, this is easier said than done, but it is doable. In fact, because a secure base can be an idea as well as a person, people, or places, the knowledge of terministic screens and the Positive Outlook could serve as a kind of secure base, itself. Knowledge of our tendencies to select and deflect could inform our every interaction and better ensure productive and generative interactions with those with whom we disagree. In this sense, we do create our own realities, and nothing, really, is forcing us to select the negative over the positive.

I believe these ideas can go a long way in improving how we talk to each other. Of course, if we are to help the world communicate better, we must practice what we preach. Although I acknowledge the difficulty in embracing the concepts discussed in this essay, I am dedicated to putting them into practice and exemplifying the kind of communication we need to grow as a society. Ideally, we can all be each other's secure base.

Author Spotlight
Erec Smith, Ph.D.

D r. Erec Smith is an associate professor of rhetoric at York College of Pennsylvania. His research includes 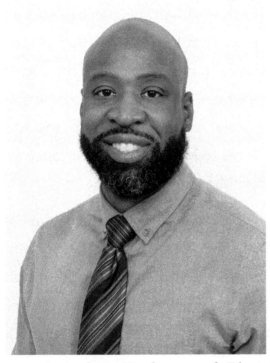 political rhetoric, size acceptance activism, workplace and social media bullying, and the confluence of rhetoric and Buddhist philosophy. His recent work focuses on the importance of empowerment and emotional intelligence in communication.

Associate Professor of Rhetoric at York College of Pennsylvania

Associate Director of the Institute for Civic Arts and Humanities

Past Chair of the York YWCA Racial and Social Justice Committee

Politics Lost: My Campaign for Office
Stacey Duckworth

I'd worked administrative positions in the health care industry for years. I'd been able to see systems, introduce systems, and help people transition to them and understand them. That knowledge allowed me to help the organization I was with run more efficiently. At the same time, I'm a people person, a good connector. When I saw that there was an open clerk position in my local government, I ran for it. I wanted to take my experience and be part of something larger than myself.

I'd never run for office before, but this wasn't an elected position as I thought of it. I would be an office manager, overseeing a department of trained admin staff. I'd use my eye for efficiency to see if and where there was a problem, and I'd make those reports and help where I could.

Maybe if I could help the court system save money and run more efficiently, it would positively impact those going through it. Maybe my small effort could help address poverty on some level. Even if not, people would see compassion when they came in front of me.

So if the election would be based on my office management skills, I'd be a natural and would win in a landslide. Easy.

Politics are rarely easy.

I was the only Democratic candidate running against three Republican candidates. I'm not even a far-left candidate. In fact, many of my supporters were Republican. I was determined to work with both sides of the aisle.

I didn't win. I lost to the son of another politician in my county where party matters more than experience. I knew my campaign would be a hard road. Even so, I still didn't realize just how hard it would be. And all during my campaign, I believed I could win.

One of the best things about my run were the wonderful people who shared space on the ticket with me. It does take a village to raise a child, and I had two in elementary school that could not be neglected. I needed a village to help me raise funds to run, to knock on doors, to call voters, to be in all the places a candidate needed to be at once. I was running for office with some extraordinary women who were on the ballot for judge, for commissioner, for city council. A few good men were on the ballot, too, and it was nice to be able to pass out one card with all the candidates from our party listed. To share event booth fees. To be hosted for fundraisers. Even with that wonderful village, the campaign was still over-whelming and I was often lonely.

I started out well. I had a support system in place. I was training for a half-marathon. I was excited to be living a life with such clear vision and purpose.

However, those last four to five months of the campaign were grueling. My carefully planned out eating and exercise routines from the beginning of the campaign evaporated. It was my final sprint to the finish line, I told myself. It would all be worth it once I pushed through and broke that finish line ribbon by being elected.

But then I wasn't. The election was over and I had lost. Having to reconcile with feeling so certain and then having the rug pulled out from under me led me to question everything I thought I knew about myself. Maybe I wasn't as good as I'd thought. My inner dialogue was on fire with self-criticism.

I was fortunate to still have a job, albeit not the one I had spent so much time campaigning for. Taking stock of the good things in hard times can be so important. That support that I'd had – including the 25,000 people who'd voted for me – that wasn't nothing and that wasn't going away, even if it didn't help calm the critical voices in my head.

I knew I needed to heal with a lot of inner work. I adopted a meditation practice, and now meditate twice a day. I also adopted a yoga practice. My inner work has taught me that I can't always make sense of a non-sensical situation. In those times, calm and clarity will come when I accept what I cannot change. Radical acceptance brings me some peace, even as I know I am still being called to make some changes in my life and the world I intend my children to grow up in.

After the election, after licking my wounds and doing the growing that I needed to do, I can say that I see things differently. I've learned to be more selective with my time and prioritize what's really important.

I recently landed a new full-time job that I think will help me learn new skills should I run for office again. If I do, I'll be smarter about some things. The experience of last campaign and the mindfulness practice I adopted after will make me a stronger person and that will make me a better candidate. I haven't thrown my hat back in the ring yet. I have big plans to see through with the members of the CHI board and I'm really excited about all that we are going to accomplish this year. But four years from now? I think you'll see my name on the ballot again. I want to be the change I want to see in the world. I'm willing to take on the next marathon.

Author Spotlight
Stacey Duckworth

Stacey Duckworth is a York County native who has discovered her passion for healing. Over the past several years, Stacey has worked to share her love of holistic approaches with her community.

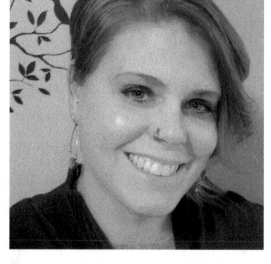

She has recently undertaken the development of CHI of Central PA, serving as president of the organization.

Duckworth works diligently to bring holistic practitioners together. She explores new avenues to bring these arts to the general public. In addition to her responsibilities with CHI, she continuously attends conferences, classes, and seminars in order to best serve her holistic community.

She is very passionate about educating the public, integrating holistic practices and connecting businesses and practitioners with each other and society members where they can be best utilized.

224

Prince Was Right
Nicole Montanarelli

Since you were born however long ago you have had titles and roles placed upon your brow. You were a son or daughter, male or female, child, friend, student, teacher, mother, uncle, discoverer, searcher, doctor, painter, fraud, military vet, etc. Every day as you grew you were given another title, another aspect of who you were to this society. These roles and titles became more distinguished as your personality took hold.

Maybe you were referred to as kind, strong, pushy, easy going, reactionary, gifted, spiritual, conforming, freaky, etc. So now you have multiple labels to describe the human form you have found yourself in. On top of all of that you also have the physical attributes of who you are fed into your mind. You are pretty, striking, fat, thin, athletic, ugly, normal, nothing special, you have a pretty face, chubby, busty, etc.

Over time you might have tried to change some of these attributes. You dieted to lose weight, you lifted heavy to become strong, you practiced your dialogue to become kinder or maybe more decisive, you had surgery to enhance or to lessen some part of you, you studied one thing feverishly to become brilliant in that way. You might have changed careers, changed roles: no longer single now a partner. You might have decided your gender was going to be more reflective of how you felt or your spouse was no longer the love you thought they were. You may have chosen to no longer act on your addictions or your fears.

There are many ways we can control what we present to the world and utilizing these options are a right we have as humans. We are searchers, all of us. We are looking for the truth of who we are. We are looking to show that truth to the world. We want others to see our truth. The act of self-discovery is often undertaken because it is time to grow. We no longer feel comfortable in the roles and titles we have been working within. They stifle us and make us feel claustrophobic. "Is this all?" we ask. So maybe we change something else. Maybe we change our hairstyle, our clothing, our religion, our daily habits. We just keep making changes until something fits...for now.

Dearly Beloved

The truth is that we are none of these labels and we are none of these roles. We choose these things, like a mask or a costume to move through our world with more ease. If you want to really know yourself, know your truth, then you have to be ready to strip away all of these things that make you, **you**.

It takes becoming okay with no longer being so much of an individual. Your pure consciousness is the same as mine, as your mother's, as your enemy, as Hitler. Your animating force is the truest version of who you are. It has absolutely no filter, no personality, no needs. Pure consciousness is just the bliss body. It is the experience of the experience being the experience.

Now, this pure consciousness was born into a human with a color, a gender, a predisposition towards certain things. All of these things we are born into are to create the experience that pure consciousness wants to have at this time.

If you were born a Saudi Prince with riches beyond compare acquired and you was the experience wanted to have. if you were born a

> **We are gathered here today...**

and all your dreams die that way, this **you**, the deep **you**, Same could be said bigot, killing people because you do not like their face. This was the experience pure consciousness needed.

It works almost like a video game of sorts, you were born a certain way, maybe your environment (that pure consciousness chose to be born into) helps to mold you, maybe your personality is a power, maybe your looks are a power...you have this video game loaded and now you have to play, with the hand you are dealt. Pure consciousness stacked the deck for you, now go experience life in this form as this player. This is where free will steps in. Yes, you are in the game, but free will allows you to follow the path so obviously laid out or you can choose to have another version of this same experience.

Be the bigot. Then go to college where you meet a young person of a different nationality and become friends. You will experience what is it like to be an ex-bigot.

Be the Saudi Prince with all the money anyone can imagine. Then decide you want to share the wealth or grow the wealth or leave the royal way...and be that experience.

The truth is that your human form will live and experience and grow **...to get through this thing...** and then, it will die. Then, pure consciousness will manifest itself into another game and the experience will be different still. The truth of who we are is that we are all just the same thing trying to play our own version of this game. We are powerful beyond measure because we can chart a reality that suits our desires.

One of the ways we can navigate this reality is to remember that everyone is playing their own version of the game. None of these human forms' experiences is the same. Everything they see or speak is unique to them. None of these human forms are conditioned into the same thing or will have the same exact life from the same exact circumstances.

We can see this when we look at siblings brought up in the same home, with the same family, same DNA, same society. For all the similar nature and nurtures, very different outcomes — looks, personality, experiences — all different. These siblings were born to play their own game.

Pure consciousness chose what deck that it would be stacked with: the looks, the likes, the visions then the siblings played. So, what is reality? Nothing really.

Birds see this world in many more colors than we do, bats use sonar to see, blind people have a different way

> **...called LIFE.**

of navigating the game, as do people born into the ghetto or into a war-torn culture or into Beverly Hills. All of these realities are very different with just enough commonalities to bring cohesiveness to our shared experiences.

Judgment is a human tool, discernment is a human tool, morality is a human tool to navigate our shared experiences that are so vastly different in this game. Yet who we are, what we **really** are, that pure consciousness is exactly the same.

Lately it is easy to notice how we are different, how we are processing differently, how we are feeling differently...it's **awakening** to our own reality. This can be a way towards magical growth as beings. Yet it can also cause us to become so divisive that we lose the one thing that ties us all together. We are all made of the same thing. Our inner truth is *exactly* the same. We are all playing our game. Our uniquenesses were given to us to be our game piece, but each of us, as a player, is the same being.

We are becoming aware of our individuality while holding strong to our awareness of the truth. We are all one. We are all playing our game. But we are all just playing and when our game ends (and it will), we will play again, differently, with different powers and scenarios. Then it will all go on again.

By choosing to see everyone you meet as another player in the game, doing what they do to experience this life, we can stop harshly judging everyone's angles. We can find ways to connect, to learn from and to appreciate the other players in this game of life. Then we play our game, the best we can and with all our powers. We do not win this game; we just get through it and onto the next.

Yoga Routine for Strength and Stamina
Nicole Montanarelli

1. mountain pose
2. sun salutation (1 round)
3. chair
4. awkward chair
5. chair
6. twisted chair
7. chair
8. twisted chair
9. chair
10. forward bend
11. high lunge
12. forward bend
13. high lunge
14. forward bend
15. side angle
16. warrior 2
17. down dog
18. side angle
19. warrior 2
20. forward bend
21. mountain pose
22. warrior 1
23. warrior 3
24. mountain pose
25. eagle
26. mountain pose
27. eagle
28. warrior 1
29. warrior 3
30. down dog
31. dolphin
32. forearm plank
33. plank
34. side plank
35. plank
36. side plank
37. locust
38. bow
39. bridge
40. reverse plank
41. twist (1 leg)
42. knees to chest
43. twist (both legs)
44. corpse

Author Spotlight
Nicole Montanarelli

Don't just survive through this life! Thrive! Utilize lifestyle changes to explore a life that is present, full and keeps you connected to yourself, others, the world, and all that is around you. Nicole is an E-RYT 500 hour yoga teacher and a YACEP 500. She holds a BS in Natural Health and Healing and is a Priest in the order of Melchizedek. Nicole is also a yoga therapist graduating from Spanda Yoga Therapy and has been practicing yoga since she was 15 years old.

Nicole has always been called to serve. She loves to work with people to offer a better way of living for themselves and a healthier way to relate to the world around them. An avid practitioner of yoga and a veracious appetite for esoteric wisdom has led her on the path of a yoga teacher, reverend and wellness coach.

Offering yoga, spiritual counseling, natural health and healing, and yoga therapy, Nicole only wishes to assist you on your own healing journey. Wake up the healer within and unite your mind, body and soul through yoga and ritual and lifestyle changes with Nicole as your guide!

Get in touch at:

Life Thrive Yoga
411 New Park Road,
New Park, Pennsylvania 17352

717 683-6284 (Nicole)

Nicole Montanarelli
lifethriveyoga@gmail.com

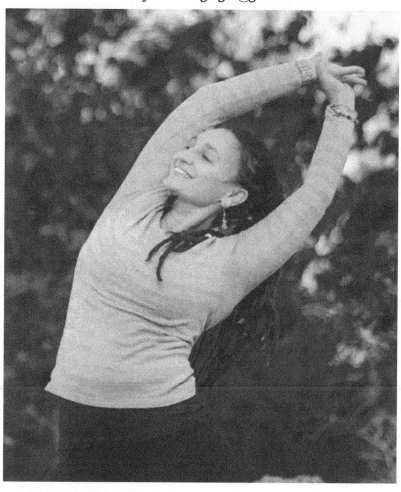

What Might Your Pets Have to Say?
Leslie Dull-Runkle

Animal communication can be used to answer all questions about your pets and even wildlife. Common questions are happiness and quality of health. Animal communication can assist in early detection and the narrowing down of the issues. This works in harmony with veterinary care. Nutritional matches can be made for optimal food choices for pets. Does your pet want a playmate? Animal communication can answer that as well as help select a compatible companion.

When a pet owner feels like they've tried every possible way to correct a behavior issue, the answers come right from your pet with animal communication. Finding lost pets and guiding you back together is animal communication. When our beloved pets seem ready to cross, animal communication assists the human with decision making. After our pets have crossed and a human would like to check in, animal communication will assist in getting questions answered.

Tuesday, November 19, 2019, I was contacted by Jolene. Henry broke from a pack with his brother Howard while on a hunting trip. Being Beagle brothers, they were noses to the ground and on the move! Jolene was in despair over Henry's great adventure with Howard. She contacted me with their story. She answered all my questions, sent me photos, then waited for my game plan. I sat quietly and connected with my two adventurers. Yes, they were safe. Yes, they were together. I knew we had a challenge on our hands. These two explorers were not having much to do with listening to me!

Jolene and I spent Tuesday, Wednesday, and part of Thursday text messaging. She was eager to confirm everything I saw and reported. Jolene knew I was one hundred percent invested in getting the boys home. She was one hundred percent invested in doing everything I asked of her.

On Wednesday, Howard had enough of the road trip. He showed up at a farm and was quickly reunited with his family. Henry, however, wasn't quite ready. Jolene was weary. I continued to encourage and support and encourage. I knew he was getting tired, wanted his human sister and all the comforts of home. Thursday he was spotted by a lady on a horse farm. This woman was as invested in getting Henry home as we were. Before Jolene headed out to the farm, I text her, "Let's bring him home."

To tell you how many trails and fields I plodded through with these two adventurers would be tough to estimate. I went to Henry and looked at the horse farm with him. We talked about the nice lady there and that she had good treats. That she was kind and loving. That Mommy was coming. Whoosh!!! I got him moving in the right direction! I received one of the best text messages of my life. It was Jolene! "Leslie, I have him!"

I cried tears of joy Thursday, November 21, 2019. Both Howard and Henry were home, safe with their families!!!

Author Spotlight
Leslie Dull-Runkle

Leslie Dull-Runkle is co-owner of Etheric Connections in Gettysburg, PA. She is a Crystal Shepherd, Animal Communicator, Usui Reiki Master, Master Angelic Light Weaver, Axiatonal Alignment Master and Priestess in the Order of Melchizedek.

She had a vision of opening a crystal shop in April of 2018. After opening the door by leaving her former job, the Universe showed her the way. That vision has today expanded to include a variety of metaphysical and spiritual tools and services.

https://ethericconnections.com
(717) 968-4241

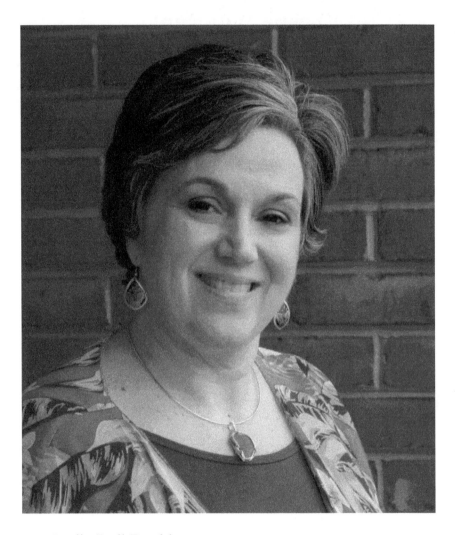

Leslie Dull Runkle
Etheric Connections

Mustard Stains and Crooked Tiaras
Phyl Campbell

In my book, *Confessions of a Grammar Enthusiast,* I saved the last essay to talk specifically about mistakes. Do we notice them? Do we point them out if asked? Do we try to hide them, or do we allow our freaky little freak flags to fly freely?

I don't know what it is about the laws of Karma, but it does seem like someone stains their shirt at any group gathering. Those of us already predisposed to feelings of nervousness or anxiety must navigate whether the bubble wrap we would cocoon ourselves in looks sillier than the inevitable food stain our clothes are likely to attract. On the opposite end, tiaras places on heads say "Look at me! Look at me!" But when a tiara is lop-sided, or placed crookedly, it sends a different message. Perhaps we are just playing dress-up. Perhaps this crown is not made for us. Combine a mustard stain and a crooked tiara and either you have an adorable five-year-old as the life of the party or an adult who is an absolute mess and possibly in need of professional help.

Even as healers, it can be difficult to get out of our own ways sometimes. Just because we decided to help other people doesn't mean we are excused from our own crap. It can help us to recognize that most people are so busy trying to hide **their** crap that they honestly don't notice ours.

By focusing our attention outward, on other people, we can help them improve. Their gratitude or signs of healing will help us in our own struggles. At the same time, one of the great services we can provide is allowing others to help us improve. Humbling ourselves to receive help is a great act of grace. When we can act with the grace we are given, we hold enormous worlds of wisdom.

Not everyone, however, is ready for our wisdom. This calls to mind the medical ethics phrase, "first, do no harm." I think that goes to the matter of mental and emotional health. When someone asks whether they look OK, or have a noticeable stain, we desire both to be kind and to be honest. It is difficult to simultaneously offer the contradictions. This feeling is exacerbated when we are asked to give an opinion by someone we do not know well. The random stranger in the dressing room doesn't trust her gaze in the mirror – but she trusts us, in that opportune moment, to be kind without leading her to embarrass herself in the harsh realities of the greater world we live in.

In these times, it is best that we ask the person what they are looking for. "If I offer my opinion," we ask her gently, "what is in your power to change?" This gives the advice seeker permission to keep the final decision for themselves. A stain might be addressed with a laundry pen or a change of clothing close at hand. An article of clothing in a dressing room might not be bought, or may be outfitted differently – a new size, a different style that is more flattering to the figure.

Another tip is to separate the person from the thing. Critique the thing, and not the person. "That shirt doesn't flatter your figure." Clearly, it's the shirt's fault, not the person's. "Hold on, your tiara is crooked." There is nothing wrong with her head. The tiara is at fault. "There, much better."

If there is nothing to be done — no laundry pens, no cute flower napkins that can cover a stain, no magical changes of clothes — then feel free to assess the situation. How bad is the stain, really? Reassure the person that anyone giving harsh judgment over a stain at a party doesn't know how to deal with life's ups and downs. Those sitting in judgment lack compassion or appropriate coping mechanisms. People with the fortitude to carry on, even to enjoy themselves, despite an imperfection, show mental wellness, perseverance, and healthy coping skills. We should all endeavor to keep mustard stains and crooked tiaras from ruining our good time.

In the written world that is my domain, asking the budding or even the experienced author — "What did you wish to convey?" — allows them to tell me about the ideas they want to get across to their readers. Their stories are quite literally theirs to tell, and anything I do must enhance the voice that they share with no one else.

We struggle. We are all imperfect and hopelessly flawed. So whenever possible, we discreetly adjust our sisters' (and all our friends') tiaras. We conspicuously ignore those errant mustard stains. We embrace imperfection while striving towards better worlds filled with better, more compassionate selves.

Author Spotlight
Phyl Campbell

P hyl Campbell, a native of northwest (the geographic location in, not a city of) Arkansas, who currently resides in York, Pennsylvania, writes fiction. And non-fiction. And basically whatever floats her boat. She hates writing her own biographies, as they are either self-deprecating or just not good, and what are the chances that someone is actually going to read the biography anyway? Well, except for you. You're special. You know you've always been different. That's why Phyl likes you so much.

Her recent series, Mermaid's Revenge, focuses on the struggle of people (and Mermaids). Power is constantly in flux, and those without it must figure out how to survive in a world with rules they did not choose and that do not benefit them. The third book of the series is due to be released summer of 2020. Books in the Mermaid's Revenge series are available on Amazon, at i-ron-ic coffee shop on Philadelphia Street in York, and on her website, www.PhylCampbell.com.

In addition to writing and publishing her own books, Phyl coaches other writers and authors from conception to publication. Her youngest Amazon author was six at time of publication. A thirteen-year-old author has published five novels with Phyl and is working on a new series. A community leader created two books to spread hope, the first with over two hundred York contributors and the second with over a thousand world-wide contributors. Phyl arranged and published them both. Visit Phyl's website for a greater sampling of fifty books and clients Phyl has helped since 2011.

Information about classes, events, workshops, and special programs can also be found via the website.

Social Media Platforms

FB PhylCampbellAuthorPage/
CreativeWritingAndPublishingWorkshop/

IG/TW: phylc_author

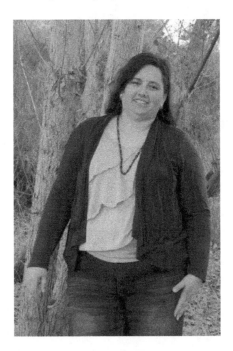

Trusting The Path
Rachel Rosado

The whole of the journey unfolds one step at a time, and in each step, we must find the trust to allow that unfolding. It's kind of like following breadcrumbs. We don't always know where we are going from the start, but if we follow that trail one crumb at a time, Spirit leads us exactly where we belong.

As a child, I saw a movie called *Resurrection* with Ellen Burstyn. Her character could heal people just by laying her hands on them and praying. Something stirred within me and I had wished then, that I might also heal others in this way. It was the first of many breadcrumbs. Later, at seventeen, I meandered into a local New Age bookstore called New Visions. I had stumbled upon a goldmine and some very eccentric yet warm and inviting gentlemen named Bill Trivett and Bob Hall. Little did I know, that they would become mentors and even spiritual guides.

I began my studies by buying three Edgar Cayce books. The first book was called *There is a River* by Thomas Sugrue. This is Edgar Cayce's biography. I also bought Cayce's book of reincarnation. The third book was Cayce's encyclopedia that mainly focuses on his readings of others' health concerns. After reading these, I went back for more and found an array of spiritual subjects that grabbed my attention. As I got to know Bill and Bob, I learned that Bob was a massage therapist. Bob gave me my very first massage and from there, massage piqued my interest.

The Baltimore School of Massage offered a five-hundred-hour program for which I was able to arrange payments. Upon graduating, I began working in a nail salon part-time. As my clientele increased, I was able to build an outcall business by word of mouth, taking my table to clients' homes.

So much joy was found in the work I was doing that I wanted more education. In 1995, this want drew me to the Cayce/Reilly School of Massotherapy in Virginia Beach, Virginia. The second day in attendance I knew I wanted to become a teacher there. The education was vast. The school is part of a non-profit organization called the Association for Research and Enlightenment or the A.R.E. They have the third largest metaphysical library in America, and host conferences with speakers from around the world. It was the perfect environment in which my desire for knowledge and expansion could grow.

One Easter Sunday I was fortunate to hear Arun Gandhi, Gandhi's grandson, talk to us about his grandfather and lessons he had taught him. There was a meditation garden and the school sat on a hill overlooking the Atlantic Ocean. It wasn't like a place on earth. The energy was unbelievable, and you could hear the roar of the ocean from the porch. How could you not want to work there? So, I did! One thing fed into another and I trusted those breadcrumbs, one step at a time. I began by assisting all the instructors which afforded me the ability to learn those classes very well. After two years I was granted instructor status of the one hundred fifty hour basic Cayce/Reilly massage course.

During that time, I also enjoyed working in the ARE's therapy department as a massage therapist. I got to work with many of the employees who came for massage. Some of them were Cayce's grandchildren. Another client was an author who was writing the Dalai Lama's biography. There was a man who was working with Egyptologists who were studying the pyramids. The most significant, however, were two different gentlemen who worked together at the Atlantic University.

They were studying Mr. Cayce's readings on Atlantis and had actually orchestrated a search to find it in Bimini. They also studied Cayce's health readings for 45 years and did many client studies and trials based on the information therein. They created a group called the Meridian Institute, a group of doctors, scientists, chiropractors, and massage therapists who all work together to practice and learn from each other based on the health readings. After accepting the request to join their group, I was also asked to help their clients with some of the health applications and massage they were working with at the time. Cayce had done 9,000 health readings. There were studies done on many different diseases and illnesses with recommendations for each individual. As the readings had been proven many times over, these were the procedures we used.

At one point I had done a specific type of spinal pattern massage that is exclusive to the Edgar Cayce Massage. The Meridian Institute was impressed and had done piezoelectric testing before and after which showed substantial improvement. They asked me to teach the group. I really enjoyed being a part of it. At the same time, I also had an outcall client with Parkinson's disease. For the most part he was bedridden but was still able to be on a massage table with my help. He told me he really looked forward to the massage and how much better he felt afterward. He had taught me so much and after two years he passed on. While teaching I was fortunate to have students from every corner of the world. One particular student was a neurosurgeon. I was very lucky to be asked to do Acupressure and Reflexology in his office. We had many different kinds of medical professionals interested in learning massage therapy. This afforded me the opportunity to pick their brains as well. Truly a lot of fun as I enjoy anatomy and physiology extremely.

My experience being an instructor at the institute and interacting with the people there was amazing. It completely changed my life and taught me to trust not only in the call of Spirit but also in myself. Initially, I struggled to speak in front of a class due to being shy. The instructor that I assisted told me, "All they want is the information. They don't care a spit about you. They are here to learn," and with that in mind, I was able get out in front of them and found confidence in a calling to teach to which I hope to be returning more fully.

Learning from people who learned directly from Cayce, expanded my own way of thinking in astounding ways. Avram from Barbados, who reminded me of Mr. Miyagi, taught us Tai Chi.

"How do you become an instructor?" I asked immediately upon meeting him.

"First, you must take a class," he answered simply.

And so, I followed the breadcrumb, and signed up for the class right away. He showed me some of the specific rotations that Cayce and Riley would use with the head that I still use today.

Sandra Duggean, another Cayce student who taught hydrotherapy and diet, was an incredible inspiration. She seemed to just glide when she walked as light emitted from her soul. I felt she was there to serve as an inspiration for us all, modelling to us the impact that Cayce's teachings could have on one's life.

As part of assisting in the Acupressure Instructor's class, I learned and instructed Ba Daun Gin, a set of Qigong movements, which is what I teach in my Stretch, Breathe, Balance class along with some spinal rotations and stretches to balance the body at Artemis today. This practice later helped me to release a lot of anger and allowed me to become more resilient, handling the ups and downs of life much better. I saw a shift in my energy and in my patience, while a deep sense of what mindfulness really is and why it's valuable emerged. It taught me to slow down as well as how to use the breath to shift the energy in my physical body.

After my marriage of twelve years fell apart in response to my husband's alcohol abuse related to ongoing depression, it was this practice that helped me restore my sense of peace and connection. I had given everything I could in hopes to heal the relationship, but due to his continued decline, the separation was best.

Because I still loved him and wanted our son to have a continued relationship with him, we moved back to PA in 2008 when he was offered a job here. These events didn't necessarily feel like breadcrumbs at the time, but looking back, I can now see how even the pain has led my growth forward. I continued to offer help and support to my former husband as we sought to share the responsibility of raising our son, but in 2012 he took his own life, and though we had been separated, the loss was harrowing.

Life collapsed. The most difficult and heartbreaking thing I have ever done was to tell my son that his father had passed. His dad was his hero and his best friend. I suffered intense grief for the loss of this man whom I had loved and for the loss of the father of my child and all of the hopes for his recovery I had somehow still carried. In all of the chaos of the move and the loss, I had stepped back from my practice for a while, but after suffering a heart attack in 2013, rehab reminded me of the benefits of physical movement and I began to incorporate stretching, Qigong, and guided meditation back into my life.

My depression at the time felt like a magnet trying to pull me down, and the spiritual component of these movements allowed me to start out the day with intention to connect to that mindfulness and allow it to flow into my day, lifting me out. I rediscovered the value and at the same time reconnected to my passion for teaching and got inspired to share.

Around the same time, I was working as a band manager. I met Chad at the Guitar Spot, who introduced me to his wife, Donna Deerin Ward, the owner of Artemis. I shared with her my passion for teaching and the fact that I know the people I teach today will get benefit from this practice. It consistently brings me back to center, like a reset button to restore calm. If this helps me so much, I know that it will help others in some way... in their own way. After talking with Donna about my desire to share what I've learned, I recognized that helping others is the core of my purpose and my class at Artemis — Stretch, Breathe, and Balance — was born. Just like that, I am back to teaching, and I hope to offer more classes as I am able.

Encouraged by Bill Trivett on my return to PA, I also received my Reiki Certification and have integrated that into my massage work. Today I offer a variety of services at the Relaxing Note in Red Lion including Acupressure, Reflexology, Neuromuscular Therapy, Cupping, Hot Stone Massage, TMJ Therapy, and the castor oil pack Cayce remedy, while also teaching at Artemis, and regularly providing chair massage for York Children's Advocacy.

Reiki has deepened the way I show up in massage. I feel the Reiki energy coming through from the heart to the hands, something I didn't notice when I was using my intention of healing before. It opens a certain state of patience and mindfulness where one can stop grasping for the right method and trust the healing to happen without direct knowledge of it. Clients feel the shift and get great results.

Still growing into my work as a teacher and a practitioner, through all of these breadcrumbs (even the challenging ones) the way I am showing up in this life has evolved. Along the way, I have learned about the importance of self-care and self-love. I have learned that you must offer yourself forgiveness, and to thank yourself from time to time for just keeping your head above water and helping others when you can. I have learned that sometimes all we need is to be held and to be listened to, and that the space we can offer one another can be more than enough. I have learned to take the time to receive and above all, I have learned the importance of trust — of following those breadcrumbs even when they don't seem to make complete sense — and trusting that I will know how they fit together when the opportunity comes.

I don't particularly know where all our breadcrumbs are leading, but I know that as we get there, there will always be enough.

Author Spotlight

Rachel Rosado-
(MSG011613), Licensed Massage Therapist

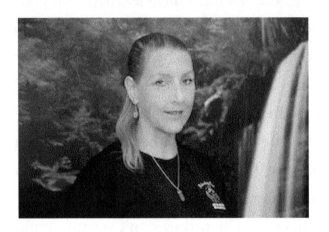

Rachel Rosado has twenty-six years of experience in the Holistic Health field and is a 1991 graduate of the Baltimore School of Massage. After graduating, she kept her own massage therapy business for four years in York, until she decided to further her studies at the Cayce/Reilly School of Massotherapy in Virginia Beach, Va. and graduated in 1996.

After becoming licensed in Virginia and board certified by the NCTMB, she became an Assistant Instructor, for two years, in the many modalities offered at the Cayce/Reilly School, including the Basic Cayce/Reilly Massage Routine, Hydrotherapy, Clinical Massage (Myofascial & NeuroMuscular), Jin Shin Do Acupressure,

Sports Massage, Intermediate Massage, Swedish, Reflexology, Therapeutic Touch, and Integrative Therapies and then became an Instructor of the Basic Cayce/Reilly routine, home remedies and diet for three years. She currently offers services through Relaxing Note in Red Lion, PA and teaches classes at Artemis- The Art of Living in Red Lion, PA. It is Rachel's goal to share the keys to balance that she has learned through her own growth journey.

Book an appointment with Rachel at Relaxing Note
141 W Broadway, Red Lion, PA 17356
717-244-1464
http://relaxingnote.com/

Check out here classes at
https://artemistheartofliving.com/

Journal Prompts
To Help You Get The Most Out of This Book

1. To which stories did you feel most drawn?

_____

_____

_____

_____

_____

_____

_____

_____

2. What feelings were expressed or issues were addressed in these particular stories?

_____

_____

_____

_____

_____

_____

_____

_____

_____

_____

_____

_____

3. What shifts were created?

_____

_____

_____

_____

_____

_____

_____

_____

_____

4. What inspiration can you take from them? Anything you could look at differently? Any encouragement or advice you can remember? Anything you can aim for yourself?

_____

_____

_____

_____

_____

_____

_____

_____

_____

_____

_____

_____

_____

_____

5. How might such a shift stand to impact your own life?
No limits! Deam **big**!

_____

_____

_____

_____

_____

_____

_____

_____

6. What do you think you need to create it?

_____

_____

_____

_____

_____

_____

---

7. Where do you think that comes from?

---

8. Do you believe you are worthy of creating such a shift in your life? You are! Write at least 3 reasons why you deserve goodness and why you know it is time!

_____

_____

_____

_____

_____

_____

_____

_____

9. Do any thoughts, practices, tools, or modalities shared in this book sound like something that may help you? (even if you create or find your own version of it)

_____

_____

_____

_____

10. Are you willing to show yourself that you deserve this shift by taking the steps to explore your path to it?

_____

_____

_____

_____

_____

_____

_____

_____

_____

11. What is one step that you can take right now?

_____

_____

_____

_____

_____

You Got This!

27 Things To Remember On Your Healing Journey

1. I have enough. I know enough. I am enough – just as I am right now.

2. I have the power to choose how I show up today. How can I use the past to grow in the present?

3. I will not blame myself for the things I didn't know, and I will seek to apply the knowledge now that I have it.

4. I deserve love and I am willing to start showing some to myself! One thing I can do to honor me is...

5. All things have light and dark. There is no good or bad. There only *is*. What judgments can I let go of?

6. In order to create change, we must first accept what we have to work with. (I call this, "MacGyver your life" LOL) What is actually here? And how can I use it to my benefit?

7. Self-care is an expression of love to all of the people with whom I interact by supporting my own capacity to engage in those interactions.

8. Growth is always available, in any situation, and I am open to it.

9. Growth isn't always comfortable, and that's okay! It's always beneficial!

10. I surrender that which is beyond my control and instead focus my energy on how to best support myself through it.

11. I am open to the rhythm, to the beauty, to the magical vibration of all that is currently here for me.

12. Emotions are not bad; they come to teach me. By allowing myself to feel and questioning where it is drawing my attention, I can learn new ways to support myself.

13. It is okay to have needs and as I become more aware of them, I am willing to speak up and accept or ask for help when needed.

14. I am creating some space and using my breath to calm down and reflect on my emotion before issuing a response.

15. I am honoring my values in all of my relationships including my relationship to myself.

16. I am prioritizing and investing my energy in accordance with my values.

17. I am an expression of Source energy.

18. My expression ripples out to impact everything. I am acting in alignment with the impact I feel called to have.

19. I am ready. I was born ready. Whole and connected, I am more than enough.

20. There are greater possibilities than I could ever imagine, and I am accepting the opportunities that give rise to them.

21. There is a rhythm to everything – ups and downs, highs and lows, ins and outs. Ease is found in accepting the flow.

22. Even when I'm feeling empty, there is always more coming in – more love, more energy, more possibility, more inspiration, more opportunity.

23. As I allow my awareness of the **more** to expand, I learn how to open myself to the abundance that *is*.

24. Inspiration is my soul speaking.

25. Self-acceptance is believing that I am worthy to receive and express that message.

26. Growth is in the allowance as I expand to authentically share my inspiration, trusting that regardless of reception, it is always *enough*.

27. Freedom is living the truth of my soul's expression.

---

*P.S. I just like the number 27. Its message is to believe in yourself, your intuitive messages, and your inner promptings. Keep doing that!

Acknowledgements

The Community for Holistic Integration would like to thank all of its members who came forth to share their stories of growth and transformation! We are proud to support such a variety of empowered Holistic Practitioners, Doctors, Energy Workers, Teachers, Artists, and Writers making a difference in our community!

Thank you also to all those who toiled behind the scenes of this project including Kimber Bowers, Phyl Campbell, Eleanor Justice, Stacey Duckworth, and to Jimmy Purkey for gracing our cover with his original artwork!

We hope that practitioners and seekers alike find hope within these pages, inspiration of how to create positive change in their own lives, and ideas of what paths to explore to support their wellness!

You can learn more about CHI and all of our local practitioners at www.chiweavers.com

Or join a supportive community of people interested in the benefits of accessible holistic healing at www.facebook.com/groups/CHIofCentralPA/

Index

A

A Place to Stand, 190, 194
Acupressure, 29, 89,90,94,248,250,252,254
Art of Living, 252
Artemis, 57, 250, 251,252,255
As Kingfishers Catch Fire, 56

B

Ba Daun Gin, 250
Baca, Jimmy, 189, 190, 191, 193,194
Baltimore School of Massage, 246,254
Belonging, 53
Body Keeps the Score, 174
Bonilla, Annabell, 106,114,119
Bowers, Kimber, 35, 44, 182, 186
Buddhism, 199,200
Burke, Kenneth, 215,216

C

Campbell, Phyl, 239, 243,266
Cayce, Edgar, 245, 248
Cayce/Reilly School, 246,254
Center of Balance, 75,80,88,92
Chaffer, Malcolm and Sue, 30
Chaya Levana. *See* Michele Lefler
Christian, 26,52,145,198
Chronister, Clint, 144, 150, 151
Church, Dawson, 159
Clark, Katye Anna, 100, 104, 105
Cognitive Behavioral Therapy, 155
Craig, Gary, 157
Craumer, Pattie, 67, 72, 73,74

D

Dewe, Bruce, 30
dis-ease, 29,66
Dispelling Wetiko, 51

doTERRA, 130, 134, 135
Duckworth, Stacey, 1, 4, 220, 224,266
Duggean, Sandra, 249
Dull-Runkle, Leslie, 234, 237
Dupes, Erika, 191

E

Eat, Pray, Love, 191
EFT. *See* Tapping
empowerment, 69, 211, 212,213,217
Energy Psychology, 164
Erato, 194
essential oils, 130, 134, 155, 157
Etheric Connections, 142,237,238

F

Felch, Linda, 62, 66,
Forder, Judy, 9, 18
Functional medicine, 96-98, 126, 132, 135, 167, 172

G

Gandhi, Arun, 246
Gilbert, Elizabeth, 191
Goal Balancing, 30
Goleman, Daniel, 213, 214,215
Green, Arlene, 29
Guitar Spot, 240
Gut Feeling, 166, 168, 169, 171

H

Hall, Bob, 245
Hample, Kerri, 94, 98, 166, 172
Healthy Living Foods, 115,116
Hermetics, 209
Hinduism, 200
Homer, 201
Hopkins, Gerard Manley, 56
Horn Farm, 55, 57
Hydrotherapy, 249, 254

Hypnosis, 40, 44, 120, 121, 122, 124

I

Illustrated Herbiary, 58
Institute of Integrative Nutrition, 129

J

Johnston, Rebecca, 126, 134
Judaism, 198, 199
Justice, Eleanor, 136, 266

K

Kalbach, Mary, 152, 161, 162, 164
Katye Anna. See Clark, Katye Anna
Kemper, Louise, 75, 79, 92
Kohlrieser, George, 211, 212

L

Lefler, Michele, 195, 203, 209
Levine, Peter, 155,156
Levy, Paul, 51
Life Thrive Yoga 233, 268
Lilienfeld, Scott, 216
limpia, 63
Lotus, 195, 200, 202
Loving Light Holistic Wellness, 45,188,268

M

mara'akame, 62,63,66
Massage, 80, 89, 90, 143, 148, 151, 246, 247, 248, 252, 254
Meditation, 22, 75, 76, 186,187, 199, 202, 203, 208, 209, 223, 247
mental health, 21, 23, 86, 96
Meridian Institute, 247, 248
mind-body, 33, 44, 132, 188
mindfulness, 80, 81, 158
Mindfulness Mentoring Institute, 164
Montanarelli, Nicole, 225, 231, 232

Movement Therapy, 157
mugwort, 57, 138
Muscle Balancing, 26, 29
Myss, Caroline, 26

N

Nature & Nourish Wellness, 131, 135
New Visions, 104, 148, 245
Nutrition 31, 116, 129, 134, 234

O

Occupational Therapy, 96, 98, 168, 172
Odyssey, 201
One Brain, 30

P

Phoenixdragonwolf, 151
Poems, 81, 86
politics, 220, 221
Positive Prime, 68-73
Powered by Your Soul, 19
psychotherapy, 26, 28, 33
PTSD, 44, 88, 107, 152-155, 159, 160
Punt, Leslie, 80, 88, 92
Purkey, Jimmy, 20, 23, 24, 266

Q

Qigong, 158, 250, 251

R

Rankin, Lissa, 159
Rebel Herbalist. See Shrader, Erin
recovery toolbox, 159
Reflexology, 80, 88-92, 248, 252, 255
Reiki, 9, 15-19, 44, 60, 75, 80, 86, 88, 92, 100-104, 142, 148, 151, 173, 174, 181, 193, 199, 209, 237, 252
Relaxing Note, 252, 255
Resurrection, 245
Rosado, Rachel, 245, 254

S

Sheehan, Kym, 191
Shrader, Erin, 5, 24, 46, 60, 61
Siegel, Dan, 159
Smith, Erec, 211, 219
Star Jaguar, 137, 138
Stewart, John, 120, 124, 125
Stokes, Gordon, 30
Stretch, Breathe, and Balance, 252
Sugrue, Thomas, 245

T

Tai Chi, 148, 249
Tapping, 28, 29, 152, 156-158, 164
Tarot, 117, 181
Tennyson, 201
There is a River, 245
Thie, John, 29, 30
Touch for Health, 28, 29, 31
Trauma, 26, 31, 36, 38, 39, 44, 56, 87,
    115, 117, 152, 155, 157, 164, 177
Trauma Recovery, 158, 160
Trivett, Bill, 245, 252

tulsi (plant), 57, 58
Turner, Toko-pa, 53, 57

V

VanBriggle, Denise, 189, 193, 194
Vanderkolk, Bessel, 155, 156

W

Ward, Donna Deerin, 251
Wetiko, 51, 53, 59
Whiteside, Daniel, 30
Wilson, Laile, 81, 85, 86,
Wixarika, 62, 66

Y

Yavicoli, Brandy, 137, 142, 143
Yoga, 60, 138, 213, 232

Z

Zimmerman, Marc, 212, 213
Zimmerman, Peg, 25, 33

CPSIA information can be obtained
at www.ICGtesting.com
Printed in the USA
BVHW040207020520
579077BV00005B/461